Natural Alternatives to Antibiotics

How you can supercharge your
immune system and fight infection

Leon Chaitow N.D. D.O.

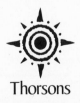

Thorsons

Thorsons
An Imprint of HarperCollins*Publishers*
77–85 Fulham Palace Road,
Hammersmith, London W6 8JB

The Thorsons website address is:
www.thorsons.com

and *Thorsons*

are trademarks of
HarperCollins*Publishers* Limited

First published by Thorsons as
Antibiotic Crisis, Antibiotic Alternatives 1998
This edition 2001

1 3 5 7 9 10 8 6 4 2

A catalogue record for this book
is available from the British Library

ISBN 0 00 712247 0

Printed and bound in Great Britain by
Creative Print and Design (Wales), Ebbw Vale

Contents

1: The Antibiotic Crisis

Crisis, What Crisis?

Health care in the industrialized world has never been more available, or so we are told.

○ More and better hospitals are built (are there more sick people?).
○ Ever more complex and high-tech treatments are devised.
○ Life-expectancy rates are rising (quantity, perhaps, but what of quality?).
○ Research continues at breakneck pace into all aspects of disease causation and treatment.
○ New, highly trained doctors and nurses are turned out every year.

…And yet there really is a crisis, as we will see.

Old diseases such as TB which were thought to be history are back, and are often untreatable because the bacterial agents which cause the infections have become resistant to antibiotics which previously controlled them easily.

This acquired resistance presents an enormous threat to the health of us all, not just those who are malnourished and impoverished.

Whether or not more and more hospitals and high-tech diagnostic and treatment methods equate with better health for the general public is itself open to question. However, what is not debatable is the fact that one of the most potent tools in the medical tool-box, antibiotics, are no longer working on many extremely dangerous bacteria, or only work when used in amounts so high that they are likely to cause serious side-effects.

The evolution of antibiotic-resistant bacteria – superbugs – therefore forms a significant part of the story we need to examine in order to understand the crisis.

The UK Office of Health Economics reported in September 1997[1] that –

○ 5,000 people are being killed every year in British hospitals by infections they catch – when they are in the hospital.
○ A further 15,000 people's deaths are being contributed to by infections they catch – when they are in the hospital.
○ One in every 16 patients who goes into the hospital for anything at all will develop a 'hospital acquired infection' (HAI) – a serious illness which they catch from someone in the hospital, usually a member of staff.
○ In intensive care units the rate is as high as one patient in every five developing an HAI.
○ The most common of the infections acquired in this way relate to the bladder, chest and surgical wounds – and many of them involve difficult to treat 'superbugs' (see below).
○ In the US, figures published in 1994 show that one patient out of every 10 develops infections caught *in the hospital*, and that this involves around 2.5 million people every year.
○ Every year 20,000 of these people die from – and the deaths of a further 60,000 are contributed to by – the hospital acquired infections, a huge number of them involving antibiotic resistant superbugs.[2]

Internal Ecological Damage

There is, however, another major outcome from the use of antibiotics which forms a less obvious but nevertheless very important part of the crisis story: the devastation that occurs in the internal environment of the body, its own ecology, especially that of the intestinal tract where hundreds of trillions of 'friendly' bacteria live and provide life-supporting services for us.

When antibiotics are used against 'bad' bacteria which infect us, these friendly bacteria are also damaged or killed. This is why major sections of this book will describe ways in which this internal ecological damage can be minimized or avoided (by using alternatives to antibiotics and improving our own natural defense systems – *see Chapters 5, 6 and 9*).

The range of conditions which can develop as a result of antibiotics causing damage to the normal intestinal flora is very wide indeed and can include:

- ○ elevated cholesterol levels – because the friendly bacteria may not be able to adequately perform their usual 'recycling' role (*see Chapter 8*)
- ○ menopausal symptoms, including osteoporosis – more likely and more severe because the friendly bacteria may not be able to perform their normal estrogen- and progesterone-recycling tasks (*see Chapter 8*)
- ○ premenstrual and gynecological symptoms – likely to be more severe for the same reasons
- ○ liver disease – more likely because the friendly bacteria may not be able to perform their normal detoxification tasks, so causing excessive loading of the liver
- ○ chronic digestive and bowel problems – because of the ecological damage caused to the normal flora, which are vital to normal digestion and intestinal function
- ○ increased risk of bladder infections – because of this ecological disorder, which allows the overgrowth of undesirable bacteria and yeasts that are often the 'reservoir' for infections in the bladder
- ○ serious arthritic conditions – can develop after antibiotic damage to the bowel flora (*for complicated reasons which are explained further in Chapter 8*)

○ depressed immune function – a not uncommon antibiotic sequel (*as explained in Chapter 5*)
○ and many, many more health problems, ranging from acne to kidney disease, can be linked to antibiotics...

The really important messages which should emerge from the discussions and evidence which will be presented in this and later chapters include the facts that –

○ Antibiotics can save lives – when used appropriately: right place, right situation, right time, right antibiotic for the correct bacteria, right amount, right means of administration (by mouth or by injection, for example), etc.
○ Antibiotics are more often prescribed 'wrongly' (*see below*) than correctly – up to 70 percent of the time, say some experts.
○ One of the results of this wrong use is the emergence of strains of bacteria which can no longer be killed by antibiotics (there are a variety of other reasons for resistance developing, as will be explained).
○ Even when used appropriately, antibiotics almost always damage the internal environment – especially of the intestinal tract – and this can itself lead to an assortment of health problems later on.
○ There are tactics, which will be explained, by means of which many of the dangers and side-effects of antibiotic use can be reduced or avoided, particularly by replenishing and revitalizing the important bacterial flora which live inside us, as explained in Chapters 7 and 9.
○ There are alternatives to the use of antibiotics; the most important of these is an efficient immune system. Methods for encouraging this will be detailed in Chapters 5 and 6.

The antibiotic crisis we face will be evaluated from different perspectives in those sections of the book which deal with protective tactics.

Natural Alternatives to Antibiotics

First it is necessary to look briefly at the individual characteristics of a selection of bacteria, as well as at the different types of antibiotics and how they are thought to work.

The 'alternatives' to the present ways of handling infection will include the use of strategies that can enhance immune function, make our natural defenses work more efficiently, and reduce toxicity, as well as ways in which damaged internal ecological systems can be repaired or improved.

After that we will survey the short- and long-term dangers of using antibiotics, descriptions will be presented, along with the evidence which supports them, by means of which we can safely reduce the hazards which antibiotics present.

The major suggestions as to what alternatives exist to antibiotics, as well as what to do if you *have* to take antibiotics (*see Chapter 9*), as well as strategies for children who have to take antibiotics (*Chapter 10*) will therefore complete our journey through the story of antibiotic use: a story of high hopes, spectacular successes, emerging doubts and finally looming disaster, as bacteria seem to be winning the battle against medical science.

There Is Real Hope

This is far from being just a doom and gloom story. We can learn a great deal from what has happened in the medical adventure which represents the story of antibiotics up till now, and this will allow us to look at alternative methods of health care and prevention, so that out of this very real crisis can come a positive change for the better.

It is necessary to repeat the statement that antibiotics can and do save lives, and probably do so tens of thousands of times every day. There are times when not taking antibiotics, or not having them administered, could prove to be an unwise, and almost certainly fatal, decision. Some indication will be offered, when we look at different forms of infection, as to when antibiotics are really necessary, and when they might be dangerous.

The crisis in antibiotic use which has gradually emerged over the past 15 to 20 years or so is only partly the result of the overuse and misuse of these potentially life-saving drugs. It is also in large part the natural (and, as we will see, not unexpected) outcome of an attack on a life-form which has found ways of protecting itself – by mutation, by natural selection, as well as by means of in-built resistance.

Resistance

Over the past 15 years a significant change has taken place in the way bacteria that cause infection respond to antibiotics. Many of the bacteria are becoming increasingly drug-resistant, so that more (and stronger) antibiotics are required to control an ever wider, and increasing, range of potentially serious infectious diseases.

As a result there are more side-effects, which are often more severe than previously, and treatment has therefore become both more dangerous and more expensive.

For example, Professor Robert Baltimore of Yale University recently reported that *Haemophilus influenzae*, which can cause meningitis and which was in the past easily controlled with ampicillin, is now (1997) resistant to antibiotics in around 20 percent of cases. They just don't work any more.[3]

The most feared superbug of all is *Staphylococcus aureus*, which has been the cause of the closure of an ever increasing number of operating rooms and hospital wards, usually temporarily but sometimes permanently, as well as being responsible for the deaths of numerous infected patients.

It has been estimated that around 90 percent of strains of *Staphylococcus aureus* are now resistant to penicillin and ampicillin, and some strains are resistant to almost all antibiotics except highly potent, highly toxic forms of antibiotic which can themselves cause serious side-effects unless used very cautiously.[4]

THE ECZEMA CONNECTION[5,6]

A new term is creeping into the medical vocabulary. Not only are we being told about the dangers of superbugs, but now there is talk of the dangers of *superantigens* (substances which provoke a severe allergic reaction). The superantigens which some bacteria can generate are being blamed for the dramatic increase in the incidence of childhood eczema.

Many bacteria do the damage they do because of toxic and allergy-provoking substances they produce. In the case of eczema, what seems to happen in an increasing number of cases is that the normal, harmless bacteria which live on the skin, such as *Staphylococcus epidermidis*, decrease in number, probably as a result of antibiotics, allowing *Staphylococcus aureus* to invade the territory usually occupied by *S. epidermidis*. This change in the local flora can cause eczema patches to become severely infected, especially if they are scratched, leading to yellow, encrusted, usually weeping lesions.

Research at the Hospital for Sick Children in London in the early 1990s showed that almost 100 percent of children with this form of severe eczema had colonies of *S. aureus* on their skin, and the more of these alien bacteria that were present the worse the eczema was. These particular strains of *S. aureus* are a new phenomenon, almost certainly resulting from changes caused by their response to antibiotics which has allowed them to produce the so-called 'superantigens'.

As Professor Bill Noble of St. Thomas's Hospital, London explains, 'These superantigens produce a horrendous response, a vicious allergic reaction at the site of the skin problem.'

Current treatment usually involves more antibiotics, steroid creams and/or antiseptic creams. Now it is reasonable to ask why, if antibiotics have helped to produce the strains of *S. aureus* which are causing this rampant increase in severe eczema, is it logical to add even more antibiotics into the picture?

This question is even more urgent when there seem to be simpler and safer answers. It has become clear that some skin specialists have found that they can deal with severe eczema without more and more antibiotics. For example, dermatologist consultants in Sheffield, England have found that they can prevent *S. aureus* from doing its damage by the simple means of abundant use of creams and oils. They explain,

> *In eczema the skin barrier is not normal, it's broken, so superantigenic exotoxins get through. But if you use plenty of emollients – bath oils, emollient creams and ointments and emollient soap substitutes (to stop the skin from drying) – you can restore the skin barrier.*

By using these and other simple techniques (including wrapping the area in wet bandages after smothering it in emollient creams), antibiotics become largely unnecessary.

The key message which this offers us is that superbugs have emerged from the inappropriate use of antibiotics, that one of the byproducts of their existence is superantigens, and that the answer (except in the short term) surely does not lie in even more antibiotics being used.

Staphylococcus aureus infection occurring in hospital settings presents us with the ultimate horror – untreatable infection. This particular superbug is the bacteria most often referred to in newspaper and magazine articles on the subject.

It is, however, by no means the only dangerous multi-resistant bacteria, and in the list in Chapter 2 a brief profile will be given of major members of this select team of bacterial antibiotic survivors, each of which has developed resistance to antibiotics and therefore has the ability to produce infections of dramatic intensity, often totally impervious to treatment.

THE 'GARBAGE CAN' EXAMPLE

Before briefly examining the superbugs, we need also to try to get a picture of an important phenomenon: the fact that many potentially dangerous bacteria (and other microorganisms) live in or on us – all the time – and do us no harm, most of the time.

The fact is that a swab of your throat or mine will reveal the presence of hundreds of different organisms, some of which are known to be involved in potentially serious infection. Among those which are almost certainly living in your nasal areas, and mine, are that most dreaded of superbugs, *Staphylococcus aureus* – so why are we not ill?

When it is functioning normally, your immune system is capable of maintaining control of these microorganisms, and prevents them from spreading and producing disease or illness. When, for any of a large number of possible reasons, your immune system operates at lower levels of efficiency, controls are weakened and this gives the microorganism the opportunity to proliferate and cause illness. For ways to boost your immune system, see Chapters 5 and 6.

The fact that for most of the time, potentially dangerous bacteria live in and on us *without causing harm*, highlights what has been called the 'garbage can' effect.

If a garbage can contains a great deal of waste which is decaying, rotting or putrefying, it will act as a magnet to flies and other scavengers who are attracted to just such material. An environment will have been created which is just right for them to use, to eat the garbage, or to lay their eggs in it perhaps.

If we create a similar environment in our own bodies, one which is 'just right' for a particular bacteria, virus or fungus, which offers it the chance to breed and eat well and where the normal controls have been relaxed, we have to expect these scavengers to take advantage of the situation.

If you were to see a garbage can overflowing with putrid material and surrounded by swarms of flies, would you be tempted to think that the problem would be solved by spraying and killing the flies? Such an approach might offer a very short-term answer to the problem, but would do nothing at all about the underlying cause as to why they were there.

Instead of trying to poison the flies, would you not consider it likely that the flies would not be there at all if the garbage can was emptied and cleaned?

The analogy in which I have compared a garbage can with an unhealthy human body is not completely accurate. However, it is true that one of the factors which can allow an explosion of activity on the part of usually inactive but potentially dangerous microorganisms in the body is a toxic state of the tissues.

A toxic condition would also involve a reduction in the efficient working of at least local aspects of the protective (immune) system, which would have been controlling the activity of bacteria, yeasts and viruses.

OPPORTUNISM

All organisms on the planet – bacteria or people – thrive if they are given the right surroundings, a condition which includes accommodation, safety from attack, adequate nourishment and a chance to breed. Therefore, if we offer bacteria, yeasts and viruses an environment in which our natural defense mechanisms offer only weak and inadequate controls, so that they will not be vigorously attacked, and if at the same time the environment (in this case part of your body) offers them surroundings which are suitable (for them) and which meet their needs – offering food and a chance to multiply – we should not be surprised if they take advantage of this. As a result, infection occurs.

And if infection occurs and involves a particular microorganism which is resistant to antibiotics, as well as being confronted by enfeebled defense systems (our immune system can become weakened for any of a number of reasons which we will explore in later chapters), we will have placed ourselves in great peril.

When bacteria (or other microorganisms) take advantage of a weak immune system, they are said to be acting opportunistically – taking their chances because they have been offered an easy ride.

The degree to which our immune system is operating efficiently or inefficiently, and the excellence, or lack of it, with which our tissues are presenting ideal, or less than ideal, conditions for potential invaders, decides how vulnerable or susceptible we are.

The comparison of this scenario with the defense of a country by its army is obvious, and as we will see in later chapters there is a great deal we can do to enhance our own personal defenses and so deny opportunities to potential enemies.

If our natural defense systems have been weakened (again, for whatever reasons) and infection threatens life itself, we need to have available options.

One choice which a suitably qualified health care provider may make in such a crisis would be to use antibiotics. But what if the organism involved is not vulnerable, has become resistant to antibiotics?

This is the scenario faced by many doctors today, often in hospital settings, where superbugs have emerged as being almost impervious to antibiotic use.

It is also happening in the community, for example as TB reappears, involving strains of bacteria which have become resistant to the medications which previously controlled them.

The ways in which this has happened will be summarized later in Chapter 2, after which we will meet some of the leading characters in the story, the superbugs.

WILL GENETIC MODIFICATION HELP?

New research has suggested that genetic engineering may allow scientists to develop ways of modifying the genetic material of bacteria such as *Staphylococcus aureus* to remove their acquired or inherited resistance to antibiotics, so once again making them vulnerable and easier to control.

In a speech to the National Academy of Sciences, Nobel Laureate Professor Sidney Altman announced that, 'This method may one day allow us to restore the full usefulness of today's front-line antibiotics.'[7]

The research which led to this statement was performed at Yale, where scientists used synthetic genetic material to 'switch off' the genes in the bacteria which produce resistance. They were in this way able to restore the sensitivity of E. coli bacteria to ampicillin, to which the E. coli bacteria had become resistant. An enormous amount of research remains to be done, most notably as to how to get the synthetic genetic material into the infecting bacteria, nevertheless this research at least offers some hope for the future.

But even if this approach proves possible and ultimately 'successful', it will only represent the continuation of a method which has led us to the present crisis situation. This is, after all, still an approach which focuses attention on 'killing the enemy' rather than improving natural defenses, which many would say was doomed to failure from the start. It is likely, therefore, that initial success in using genetic engineering on resistant bacteria to once again make them vulnerable to antibiotics is almost certain to result, in time, in these bacteria finding other ways of becoming resistant, as they have so successfully done up till now.

WHY DO BACTERIA DEVELOP RESISTANCE TO ANTIBIOTICS?

In his book *Alternatives to Antibiotics*, Dr John McKenna reports that in the early days of the use of penicillin, its discoverer, Alexander Fleming, warned that if antibiotics were used inappropriately bacterial strains would mutate to produce resistance to the drugs.[8] This would be more likely, and possibly more serious, if:

○ antibiotics (penicillin was the main one being used in 1945, when this statement was made) were used orally. By using the drug intravenously it would be more likely to reach the target area, whereas taken orally this is less certain.
○ the wrong doses were given. Too little would allow some bacteria to survive, and so increase the risks of mutation.
○ courses were not completed. This too would lead to survival of some, hardier bacteria, which would then proliferate.

○ courses went on too long. This would increase the likelihood of resistant organisms emerging from the attack on
them, as well as the probability of damage occurring to
the internal ecology of the body, something we will dis-
cuss in more detail in Chapters 8 and 9.

Clearly Fleming was correct.

And to this list should be added one of the worst of all 'wrong
uses': when an agent (antibiotic) is used to treat something it
cannot control, for example a virus.

A report in the *British Medical Journal* on research done at
Southampton University indicated that when antibiotics are
given to treat a sore throat (which could be of viral or bacterial
origin) it made no difference whatever to the time it took for
the individual to recover.

○ Over 700 patients were treated for 10 days with either
antibiotics or with nothing at all.
○ All the patients got better at the same rate.

It is common practice for doctors to issue prescriptions, often in
submission to demands by patients, for problems such as this.
Undoubtedly, the degree of such inappropriate antibiotic use
has added to the superbug phenomenon.[9]

Another study conducted in Holland involved over 200
patients with inflamed sinuses, confirmed by x-ray, in which
half the patients were given antibiotics and the other half a
dummy pill. There was no difference whatever in the speed of
recovery, or in the number of subsequent relapses as confirmed
when these patients were contacted a year later on.

Otitis media and Antibiotics

The way Otitis media (infection of the middle ear) has been and is being treated and mistreated using antibiotics gives us a perfect example of the problems we face.

Here we see a condition which is widespread, almost always bacterial in origin, almost always self-limiting (that is, gets better on its own), and almost always attracts antibiotic treatment – as a result of which resistant strains of bacteria have developed. Yet this obviously 'wrong' treatment continues to be suggested in most cases by most doctors and many specialists.

Consider what is now known (or what should now be known) about antibiotic treatment for Otitis media, which affects tens of thousands of children each year.

If your child has otitis it is very likely that antibiotics will be prescribed for a course which could run for between 3 and 10 days, depending upon what the doctor believes and has read of current research. As we will see, no antibiotics at all is usually the best choice, and if any are given 3 days is as good as 10. Along with the antibiotics, decongestant and painkilling medication will also usually be prescribed.

In the normal course of events, relief from the pain of the ear infection will be noticed by the distressed child within a matter of hours. And the grateful parent is likely to think – 'how wonderful, how good that the pain and distress is easing, bless the antibiotics' ... and yet...

As far back as the early 1970s doctors at the University of Copenhagen were recognizing that the repeated use of antibiotics to treat children's ear infections led to an increased likelihood of:

○ more ear infection and therefore more antibiotics, and
○ a greater chance of surgery ultimately being needed.

They decided that such problems should be treated in other ways.[10]

They claimed, after much research that, '88 per cent of patients [with otitis] never need antibiotics.' They had found that the frequency of recurrence of otitis media in the many children with otitis whom they were treating and who were *not* receiving antibiotics was low compared with those who were receiving antibiotics, who commonly had another ear infection within a month or so of the end of their course of antibiotics.

More recent research has validated the Danish viewpoint, with serious doubts being raised as to the usefulness (and wisdom) of antibiotic care of otitis.

These doubts have been regularly expressed in major medical journals such as the *British Medical Journal*, the *Lancet* and the *Journal of the American Medical Association*, where we might expect some notice would have been taken by those responsible for the health of our children.[11,12]

The American researchers stated, 'Recurrence rates were significantly higher in the antibiotic treated group [of children] than in the placebo group [those receiving dummy medicines].' In fact, the children receiving antibiotics were between 200 and 600 per cent more likely to have recurrence of the ear infection compared with children receiving no antibiotic treatment at all – whose own immune systems were dealing with the infections.

In 1981 a study was performed involving over 170 children with otitis. All the patients were given the usual painkilling and decongestant medicines; some were then also prescribed antibiotics, others also had both antibiotics and surgery (myringotomy – where the ear drum is punctured to release fluids which are pressing on it), while others had this form of surgery but were not prescribed antibiotics.

THE RESULTS?

There was no difference at all between any of the groups of children as far as

◯ the rate of recovery from pain
◯ how quickly temperature normalized

○ how soon ear discharge stopped

○ the appearance of the inner ear

○ the rate of recurrence of infection.

There was no difference at all whether antibiotics were given or not!

The same researchers looked at the problem again in 1985, this time involving nearly 5,000 children with otitis.[13]

This time they found that 90 percent of the children recovered, without any problems, without antibiotics, only having painkillers and decongestants to ease the symptoms while they recovered on their own.

So we see that as long ago as the late seventies and early eighties reputable scientific evidence existed showing that children who had antibiotics for middle ear infections usually did not benefit from them and were more likely to get another infection soon, compared with children not given antibiotics.

SUMMARY

○ Treating otitis with antibiotics seems to increase the chances of further infection by between 200 and 600 percent.

○ Treating otitis with antibiotics seems to increase enormously the chances of surgery being required.

○ Around 90 percent of children get better just as fast, with no significant differences in speed of relief of pain, temperature or other symptoms – whether they have antibiotics or not in treating their otitis.

○ Treating otitis media with antibiotics devastates the friendly, useful internal flora with potentially harmful bacteria and yeasts likely to replace them.

○ Treating acute otitis with antibiotics is just as 'effective' whether it lasts for 3 days or 10 days – and it is not hard to know which would do less harm to the friendly bacteria.

Antibiotic Misuse

After confirming their belief that bacteria possess remarkable abilities to mutate and defend themselves, something we can do little about at this stage, Professor French and Emeritus Professor Phillips of the Department of Microbiology at St. Thomas's Hospital, London, are scathing in their comments as to factors we *could* do something about, including the wrong use of antibiotics:[14]

> *Antibiotic misuse is common. Studies have shown that up to 70 per cent of treatment courses are 'unnecessary' or 'inappropriate'; Therapy is often unnecessarily prolonged … physicians are often poorly informed about the use of antibiotics and may obtain most of their information from pharmaceutical companies.*

They also condemn the widespread and apparently haphazard use of antibiotics in animal farming as a cause of the spread of resistance.

Aside from these elements of overuse, misuse, abuse of (and sometimes failure to use) antibiotics, the particular situations which occur in hospitals are a key factor in the evolution of resistant strains.

What we are seeing is an approach to treating infection which actually makes greater infection and general disease more likely. This approach calls into question the ability of those responsible for our health to think more than a few days' hence, since the prospects it produces of untreatable superinfections becoming rampant in the community, as well as in hospitals, is too frightening to contemplate. And, being too frightening to contemplate, it is not thought about – it is left as something which will be dealt with when it happens.

Unfortunately for the general population, it is already happening.

It is not as though warning bells have not been ringing for years:

○ Books such as Marc Lappe's *When Antibiotics Fail* were met when first published in the mid-1980s with glowing reviews in the major medical and lay press, yet nothing appears to have been done to stem the tide of misuse and overuse of antibiotics by doctors.

○ Geoffrey Cannon's major book *Superbug*, diligently researched and referenced, first appeared in 1995 and was reviewed in the popular press with words such as 'It delivers a message that will haunt the average pill-swallower for life' (*Daily Express*) and was welcomed by leading microbiologists. It does not (as yet) seem to have made much impact on medical prescribing habits of antibiotics, despite showing clearly just how serious the crisis is.

○ According to the *British Medical Association's New Guide to Medicines and Drugs* (1995), one prescription out of six is for antibiotics, and it is estimated by researchers such as Lappe that most of these are inappropriate and/or excessive, producing the perfect situation to encourage increased resistance.

Lappe discusses the frightening degree of resistance to antibiotics of *Neisseria gonorrhoea*, the organism responsible for gonorrhea, and makes the point that between 1986 and 1988 there was a 60 percent increase in resistance to penicillin, and that to cover this change tetracycline was introduced. This, too, quickly produced resistant strains, leading to the introduction of spectinomycin, which by 1988 had resulted in the first resistant strains (to it) being discovered. As a further twist in this never-ending game of catch-up, some hospital groups now use ever more powerful and expensive anti-gonorrhea cephalosporin antibiotics, such as ceftriaxone.

As Lappe sees it,

This 'new' (and expensive) therapeutic fix to a social problem may yet meet a similar fate. Unless antibiotic uses are coupled with sound health education about the hygienic

measures needed to control the epidemic, no success in abat-
ing this epidemic is likely. Just such success has been chart-
ed in the gay community, where the widespread practice of
'safe sex' has led to an abatement of both AIDS and gonor-
rhoea in California.

This important insight of Lappe's needs emphasis:

○ Unless causes are dealt with, antibiotics will fail in the long run – even if they are used sensibly.
○ If problems emerge from a lack of hygiene, then the 'cure' lies in better hygiene.
○ If causes lie in poor nutrition, then 'cure' lies in better nutrition.
○ If causes lie in poverty and social problems, then political and social action is needed – not the pumping of ever more antibiotics (or whatever) into the already sick population, an approach which simply masks the symptoms, ignores the causes and sets the scene for the infection explosion many now anticipate.
○ In the short term it makes sense to use antibiotics to save lives. But the antibiotics must be used sensibly, cautiously, appropriately and not haphazardly and excessively, as they are now.
○ Even when used correctly and appropriately (and remember, please, that Professors French and Phillips – quoted earlier in this chapter – believe that over 70 percent of antibiotics are 'wrongly' prescribed), serious long-term changes occur in our internal ecology when most antibiotics are taken, involving the friendly bacteria which keep us alive. This makes antibiotic use a potential health hazard even when prescribed and taken correctly and appropriately.
○ In the long term, underlying causes of ill-health have to be addressed both on a large scale by health authorities and government, and on an individual level by an accep-tance of responsibility – by a recognition that each of us

has the power to decide whether to maintain hygienic habits in our lives. Each of us can, if we wish, undertake to incorporate health-enhancing practices, rather than disease-causing ones, into our daily lives.

Many aspects of these health-promotion practices and immune-enhancing methods are discussed in later chapters.

What Happens in Hospitals?

○ Drugs, especially antibiotics, are widely used.
○ The presence of many different diseases and associated microorganisms offers a greater chance for cross-infection – infections being transferred from one person to another.
○ Highly specialized drugs, which may be new or only capable of being used under controlled conditions, are often used in hospitals only – so exposing bacteria to new substances to which they can start becoming resistant.
○ Antibiotics applied to the skin are widely used in hospitals and can lead to resistant strains rapidly emerging (this is something which has been observed when extensive use of antibiotics are involved in treating burns cases, for example).
○ It is common for people who spend time in the hospital – staff as well as patients – to become colonized with resistant bacteria, especially in their intestinal tracts (so allowing the bacteria to appear in their feces) and on the skin.
○ It is all too easy for staff to pass such resistant bacteria around as they touch patients, their beds or their food.
○ When catheters are used or injections given, previously harmless skin bacteria which may have been modified into disease-causing bacteria can enter through the broken skin, causing infection, sometimes extremely seriously, of the bloodstream.[15]

Natural Alternatives to Antibiotics

○ Unless scrupulous hygiene is observed, bacteria on the skin or in the feces can become the means whereby outbreaks of highly contagious resistant bacteria can take place in hospitals.

○ There exist (undetected by routine checks) highly infectious bacteria in hospital air-conditioning units, which can act to spread infection from ward to ward.[16]

Solutions lie in better hygiene and hospital organization, although to an extent the factors prevailing in these hothouses of disease management cannot easily be altered and solutions need to also involve patient and medical staff education as well as removal of the pressure exerted by drug manufacturers on those who prescribe the drugs.

Summary

Bacteria have developed resistance to antibiotics because of:

○ natural selection – genetic modification of the bacteria as they defend themselves from chemical assault

○ inappropriate and excessive use of antibiotics in food production, notably beef, milk and chickens

○ inappropriate and excessive use of antibiotics in treating humans – as discussed above

○ poor cooperation by patients (not completing courses of antibiotics, for example)

○ increased opportunities for cross-infections which allow resistant bacteria to transfer this characteristic to other bacteria, so spreading the pool of resistant microorganisms

○ increasing existence of unhygienic conditions where cross-infections become more likely (e.g. needle sharing)

○ particular characteristics prevailing in hospital environments which encourage the development of resistant strains

– as well as a higher risk of cross-infection via patient-to-patient contact, or transmitted via hospital personnel.

This book's task is to point to solutions to the crisis which is already here. Your task is to try to do something about this crisis in your own life – by learning more, trying harder to accept responsibility for enhancing your own health, and doing your best to ensure that the truth about antibiotics spreads.

People demand antibiotics, and doctors commonly comply, often knowing that taking them is worse than useless in a given situation. People who understand these dangers will help doctors to reserve the use of antibiotics to those times when they are indeed life-savers.

2: Bacteria – The Good, the Bad, and the Frightening

We have seen something of the crisis in which we find ourselves as a result of misguided use of the potentially life-saving antibiotic drugs –

- ○ because they are prescribed to treat conditions they cannot help
- ○ because they are wildly and massively overused in conditions that would get better on their own
- ○ because they are prescribed in the wrong dosage, wrong combinations (or not in combination when this would be a better strategy), wrong situations, for inappropriate lengths of time – often in the hot-house situations which exist in hospitals, the 'superbug factories'
- ○ because they are used in agriculture, animal – dairy, meat and fish – as well as some fruit production, in a staggering and seemingly uncontrolled way.

And as a result of all of these misuses of antibiotics we are witnessing the looming crisis of bacterial infections which will be untreatable.

This monster – the totally antibiotic-resistant bacteria which are being unleashed on the human and animal kingdom – will require strategies other than more and more powerful antibiotics. These strategies form much of the remainder of this book, after examining what antibiotics actually do in Chapters 3 and 4.

In this chapter we will get to know some of the cast of characters involved in this saga – those that live in and on us, at best enormously beneficial and at worst potentially disease-causing, as well as a number of the bacteria which cause disease, sometimes mild but often with the potential, in the right circumstances (right for them, wrong for us) to cause life-threatening illness.

The (Usually) Friendly Bacteria

There are actually hundreds of different bacterial organisms and many more different strains living inside us, many doing useful jobs, as we will see. However, there are only a few which are present in really large numbers, and it is these which we will now examine briefly. For further details of their functions, what can harm them and what we can do to encourage their (and therefore our) health, see Chapters 9 and 10.

There is evidence that under the appropriate conditions, some of the friendly bacteria can become dangerous to us. One such situation can occur when there has been excessive use of antibiotics. This will be described more fully in Chapter 4.

Some of the 'normal resident' bacteria described below (*S. faecalis*, for example) have a borderline status – normally they do no harm, but they have been implicated in infection – of the bladder, for example – in some cases.

We have to remember that there is a delicate symbiotic (mutually beneficial) relationship between us and the organisms that have lived inside us for millions of years, but in the end they are looking after their own best interests and not ours; we benefit from them when all the environmental conditions are as they ought to be. One of the factors which can seriously disrupt the environment in which these bacteria live is the use of antibiotics, which while killing 'bad' bacteria do harm to the 'good' ones as well (not all antibiotics do this to the same degree, as will be seen in Chapter 4).

BIFIDOBACTERIUM BIFIDUM

These friendly bacteria inhabit the intestines – with a greater presence in the large intestine (the colon) than the small intestine. They also live in the vagina. In breastfed babies together with *B. infantis* and *B. longum* they form 99 percent of the flora of the intestines, but gradually reduce in numbers as we age. Their major roles are:

○ preventing colonization by hostile microorganisms by competing with them for attachment sites and nutrients
○ preventing yeasts from colonizing the territories which they inhabit
○ helping to maintain the right levels of acidity in the digestive tract to allow for good digestion
○ preventing substances such as nitrates from being transformed into toxic nitrites in our intestines
○ manufacturing some of the B-vitamins
○ helping detoxify the liver.

LACTOBACILLUS ACIDOPHILUS

This natural inhabitant of the intestines also lives in the mouth and vagina. Its main site of occupation is the small intestine. Its major roles are:

○ preventing colonization by hostile microorganisms such as yeasts by competing with them for attachment sites and nutrients
○ producing lactic acid (out of carbohydrates) which helps to maintain the correct environment for digestion, by suppressing hostile organisms (other bacteria and yeasts)
○ improving the digestion of lactose (milk sugar) by producing the enzyme lactase
○ assisting in the digestion and absorption of essential nutrients from food

- destroying invading bacteria (note that not all strains of *L. acidophilus* can do this, however)
- slowing down and controlling yeast invasions such as Candida albicans.

BIFIDOBACTERIUM LONGUM

This is a natural inhabitant of the human intestines and vagina. It is found in larger numbers in the large intestine than the small intestine. Together with other bifidobacteria, this is the dominant organism of breastfed infants (making up 99 percent of the microflora). In adolescence and adult life the bifidobacteria are still the dominant organism of the large intestine (when health is good). Among its main benefits are:

- preventing colonization by hostile microorganisms by competing with them for attachment sites and nutrients
- production of lactic and acetic acids, which inhibit invading bacteria
- helping in weight gain in infants by retention of nitrogen
- preventing harmful nitrites being formed from nitrates in the digestive tract
- manufacturing B-vitamins
- assisting in liver detoxification.

BIFIDOBACTERIUM INFANTIS

This is a natural inhabitant of the human infant's digestive tract (as well as of the vagina, in small quantities). Its presence is far greater in the bowel of breastfed infants compared with bottle-fed infants. Among its main benefits are:

- preventing colonization by hostile microorganisms by competing with them for attachment sites and nutrients
- production of lactic and acetic acids, which inhibit invading bacteria

○ helping in weight gain in infants by retention of nitrogen
○ preventing harmful nitrites being formed from nitrates in the digestive tract
○ manufacturing B-vitamins.

LACTOBACILLUS BULGARICUS

This extremely useful friendly bacteria is not a resident of the human body, but a 'transient'. Once it enters the body through food (yogurt, for example) it remains for several weeks before being passed, but while in the body it performs useful tasks. *L. bulgaricus* is a yogurt culture, as is the other main yogurt-making culture, *Streptococcus thermophilus* (*see below*), and is therefore found in some yogurts and cheeses if they have not been sterilized to kill their bacterial cultures – to enhance shelf-life – after manufacture. It performs a number of useful roles, such as:

○ Some strains produce natural antibiotic substances.
○ Some strains have been shown to have anti-cancer properties.
○ They enhance the ability to digest milk and its products by producing the enzyme lactase, which is absent or deficient in almost half the adults on earth, and many children, especially if they are of Asian, African or Mediterranean descent.
○ Because they produce lactic acid (as do all bacteria with 'lactobacillus' as the first part of their name), they help to create an environment which encourages colonization by the bifidobacteria (they are therefore known as 'bifido-genic' bacteria) and by *L. acidophilus,* by helping to prevent colonization by other, undesirable microorganisms.

STREPTOCOCCUS THERMOPHILUS

This is a transient (non-resident) bacteria of the human intestine which together with *L. bulgaricus* (*see above*) is a yogurt culture, also found in some cheeses. It performs a number of useful roles, such as:

○ Some strains produce natural antibiotic substances.
○ They enhance the ability to digest milk and its products, by producing the enzyme lactase.
○ They produce lactic acid, thereby helping to create an environment which encourages colonization by the bifidobacteria and by *L. acidophilus*, and which discourages colonization by other, undesirable microorganisms.

STREPTOCOCCUS FAECIUM

This is a natural resident of the human intestine. It is found in human feces as well as on some plants and insects. Its characteristics include:

○ It is used as a part of the manufacture of cheeses (in some dairies, not all).
○ Its potential benefits to humans remain a possibility but not a certainty.
○ It manufactures lactic acid from carbohydrates and so enhances the environment for colonizing friendly bacteria.

STREPTOCOCCUS FAECALIS

This is a resident of the human intestine which is known as an enterococcus. It is found in feces, some insects and some plants. Its characteristics include:

○ the manufacture of lactic acid from carbohydrates, thereby enhancing the environment for colonizing friendly bacteria

○ the production of substances called amines, which can be toxic. Tyramine, for example, is associated with migraine headaches, and histamine with allergic and inflammatory reactions.
○ has been associated with urinary tract infections
○ overall there is little evidence that *S. faecalis* is beneficial for humans; on balance it would seem to have a harmful potential.

Some additional (usually useful) lactobacilli found in the digestive tract include:

○ *L. casei* – a transient bacteria of the intestine, found in cheese and other dairy products; manufactures lactic acid, so reducing the chances of invading bacteria being able to colonize the area
○ *L. plantarum* – a transient bacteria of the intestine, found in dairy products, sauerkraut, pickled vegetables; manufactures lactic acid
○ *L. brevis* – a transient bacteria of the intestine, found in dairy products (especially kefir, a fermented milk drink); manufactures lactic acid
○ *L. salivarius* – a natural resident of the mouth and digestive tract; manufactures lactic acid
○ *L. delbrueckii* – a transient bacteria of the intestine, found in grains and vegetables which have been fermented; manufactures lactic acid
○ *L. caucasicus* (known as *L. kefir*) – a transient bacteria of the intestine, found in kefir grains and drinks; manufactures lactic acid (as well as alcohol and carbon dioxide). It therefore inhibits undesirable bacteria.

The Not-so-friendly Bacteria and the Superbugs

The prospect of control over superbugs lies in the future; for the present we need to have a degree of understanding and awareness of the nature and potentials of the major antibiotic-resistant microorganisms.

STAPHYLOCOCCUS AUREUS

This bacterium is present in almost everyone, usually living in the nose. It is commonly involved in infections of

○ the skin (boils and abscesses, for example)
○ conjunctiva of the eyes (conjunctivitis).

When it has entered the body, often in a hospital, possibly after surgery, it can be the major cause of infections of:

○ the lungs (pneumonia)
○ the brain (meningitis)
○ the bones or bone marrow (osteomyelitis)
○ the heart (endocarditis).

Or it can be involved in some horrendous, often fatal, conditions such as:

○ Toxic Shock Syndrome
○ Scalded Skin Syndrome (SSS), in which the skin sloughs off the body as though it had been burned.

In both SSS and Toxic Shock Syndrome there seems to be a combined involvement of *Staphylococcus aureus* and a potentially dangerous yeast, *Candida albicans* (which lives in everyone on the planet, usually harmlessly). Candida often proliferates in the intestinal tract after antibiotic use, when its natural controls, including the flora of the bowel, are damaged.

Dr. Eunice Carlson of Michigan University has shown that when Candida is actively present in the system at the same time as an infectious agent such as *Staphylococcus aureus*, the toxic effects of *Staphylococcus aureus* are hugely enhanced and can result in fatal Toxic Shock Syndrome.[1]

As time has passed, *Staphylococcus aureus* has become resistant to almost all antibiotics apart from Vancomycin, which is now used specifically for the purpose of controlling it.

Vancomycin has potentially dangerous side-effects, is difficult to administer (usually via a drip) and is costly. This is the only remaining *Staphylococcus aureus* antibiotic. If resistance to vancomycin also develops, as is almost certain in time, there are no other antibiotic treatment methods currently available.

Other commonly resistant (to antibiotics) staphylococci include *Staph. epidermidis* and *Staph. haemolyticus*. Widespread, hospital-acquired infections involving these bacteria are now commonly treated with vancomycin, although this is often an inappropriate means of controlling them, according to leading experts.

As Professor French and Emeritus Professor Phillips, both of the Department of Microbiology at St. Thomas's Hospital, London, say, 'These infections often do not require antibiotic therapy, and unnecessary use of vancomycin for these organisms may be one factor in the emergence of ... resistance.'[2]

They believe that as these staphylococci acquire resistance to vancomycin they may be able to transfer this to the far more dangerous organism *Staphylococcus aureus*. Were this to happen, these researchers state, 'Serious, untreatable staphylococcal infection would result.'

Once again we see, despite all the warnings that have been given, as well as the experience of the past, that inappropriate treatment is being used, with potentially disastrous consequences in store. Particular antibiotics are being used where they should not be used, and as a result resistance is likely to grow to the one antibiotic that can still control *S. aureus*.

CORYNEFORM BACTERIA

These bacteria are normally harmlessly present on almost everyone's skin. In most cases they are sensitive to antibiotics. However, in hospital settings patients often become colonized with resistant strains and species which can then cause infections – if there is an opportunity, something far more likely in hospital settings, for any number of reasons including the obvious one that people in the hospital are more prone to having lowered immunity because they are already ill.

Infection with *Coryneform Bacteria* is most common where catheters and prostheses are involved, or in patients whose immune systems are struggling because of various blood-related and malignant diseases.

In hospitals *Coryneform Bacteria* are now resistant to most antibiotics and respond only to vancomycin.

STREPTOCOCCUS PNEUMONIAE

These bacteria, as their name suggests, are often involved in pneumonia, but they may also cause meningitis and are often associated with infections of the sinuses, ears, blood, and lungs.

When only low levels of resistance are found in the bacteria, high doses of penicillin will still control infections in which they are involved. However for those strains which have developed resistance to many antibiotics the treatment commonly involves the powerful drug vancomycin, or a cephalosporin antibiotic such as cefoxtaximine.

Researchers note that there are now signs that this last-mentioned class of drugs are gradually losing their power to control the bacteria, and there are major fears that this resistance will increase over time.

ENTEROCOCCI

These organisms live mainly in the bowel and may become involved in infections of this region. They can also cause infections of:

○ the blood (bacteraemia)
○ the heart muscle (endocarditis)
○ the urinary tract
○ the endometrium in the uterus.

They are frequently involved with infection associated with the use of catheters (obviously something more likely to be happening in the hospital than anywhere else), as well as in peritonitis.

In hospital settings the particular bacteria from this group which are most commonly found to be involved in serious infection are *Enterococcus faecalis* and *Enterococcus faecium*. The latter, which in the past has been considered relatively unimportant and not dangerous (and easily controlled), is now found to be increasingly resistant to most antibiotics.

To quote Professors French and Phillips, 'These organisms are among the most important and problematic multidrug resistant pathogens of the 1990s.'

HAEMOPHILUS INFLUENZAE

This is frequently associated with infections of the:

○ throat
○ sinuses
○ ears
○ bones and joints
○ chest
○ meninges of the brain
○ and sometimes breast infections in women (mastitis).

This organism has gradually increased its resistance to the major drugs used to control it, including ampicillin. In one major incident in Spain in the early 1980s, resistance was demonstrated to chloramphenicol and ampicillin by around 60 percent of *Haemophilus influenzae* strains found in patients with meningitis.

It is, however, still very susceptible to antibiotics such as cefuroximine and cefaclor, although even in these a small degree of resistance is now being reported.

NEISSERIA GONORRHOEA

This organism is involved in:

○ sexually transmitted diseases such as gonorrhea
○ pelvic inflammatory disease
○ some eye infections, and
○ sore throats (rare), often when there is also genital infection.

Neisseria gonorrhoea is now widely resistant to penicillin-type antibiotics and also, increasingly, to tetracycline. At the moment it is demonstrating only slight resistance to commonly used antibiotics such as spectinomycin and fluorinated quinolones.

NEISSERIA MENINGITIDIS

This is involved in:

○ bacterial meningitis infections
○ acute sore throats.

For many years sulfonamide drugs were used to treat infections caused by *Neisseria meningitidis;* however in the 1960s resistance developed which made this form of antibiotic relatively useless. It was however still (and remains) largely controllable by penicillin, although this too is beginning to change.

Just how rapidly resistance to antibiotics can develop is illustrated by the pattern found in Spain, where in 1985 *Neisseria meningitidis* was not at all resistant to penicillin. However, by 1987 approximately 7 percent of the organisms were showing resistance, and by 1989 20 percent had reduced susceptibility to penicillin.

ENTEROBACTERIA

This group includes *E. coli*, *Klebsiella*, *Enterobacter*, *Serrata* spp, *Shigella*, *Salmonella* and *Campylobacter*. These organisms are found in almost everyone's intestinal tract, in small numbers. It is when changes occur which allow them to become rampantly infectious that problems arise – once again we see how important the environment in which bacteria live is to how they behave, and must keep reminding ourselves that the 'environment' of the intestinal tract, above all other parts of the body, is capable of being seriously damaged when antibiotics are used.

The enterobacteria can be involved in infections of the:

○ intestinal tract, for example in food poisoning
○ abdomen (often following injury; also in peritonitis)
○ ear (acute otitis media)
○ blood (bacteraemia)
○ bones and joints
○ brain (often in brain abscesses; in meningitis of newborn babies)
○ tissues under the skin (cellulitis; a potentially very serious infection, often as a result of intravenous drip insertion)
○ some eye infections
○ lungs (pneumonia) and, not uncommonly,
○ infections involving transplant patients.

Many of these organisms are now resistant, to a greater or lesser degree, to a range of antibiotics. For example, *E. coli* (a common food poisoning agent), although usually sensitive to ampicillin and amoxycillin, has occasionally shown multiple resistance to almost all antibiotics, and this trend is expected to continue.

Klebsiella, Enterobacter and *Serrata* spp have in the past often caused outbreaks of infection in hospitals; these outbreaks have been controlled by the use of antibiotics such as cephalosporins and aminoglycosides. Researchers report, however, that strains of *Klebsiella* have now appeared which are capable of producing serious infections, especially in people with compromised immune systems, and which have become resistant to almost all antibiotics except for carbepenems.

Salmonella, one of the enterobacteria, is often a cause of food poisoning. About 80 percent of the bacteria recovered from infected patients are found to be resistant to major antibiotics. They remain susceptible to some fluoroquinolones antibiotics, although resistance is on the increase.

Professors French and Phillips add their voices to the controversy surrounding feeding animals with antibiotics. They point out that there is strong evidence that the use of antibiotics in animal feeds (to increase the animals' growth rate) has contributed greatly to resistance in many of those enterobacteria found in human infections. This trend continues, unfortunately; as more advanced antibiotics (quinolones, *see Chapter 4*) are being used in farm settings, so resistance to these drugs has now appeared when humans are being treated for salmonella infection relating to food poisoning.

The use of antibiotics in animal production for food has been a cause of concern for many years. In 1986 after discovering that fully one-third of patients hospitalized with antibiotic-resistant infections had had no previous antibiotic treatment themselves, the Swedish government banned antibiotics in animal feed because of the fear that their use was breeding antibiotic-resistant microorganisms and that these were being transferred to humans when consumed in meat.

Since 1988 almost all Swedish farm animals are antibiotic-free, and they are also among the only commercial flocks which are free of salmonella as well.[3,4]

Natural Alternatives to Antibiotics

Unfortunately, largely because of economic factors and enormous pressure from the pharmaceutical industry, few other countries are even considering this vital step, a state of affairs which is certain to encourage the further development of antibiotic-resistant strains.

PSEUDOMONA AERUGINOSA

This bacteria is commonly involved in infections acquired while in the hospital (known scientifically as *nosocomial* infections – after the Greek word for hospital).

It is not uncommon to find it involved in infections of:

○ the blood
○ bones
○ joints
○ lungs
○ the urinary tract
○ the abdomen (peritonitis).

It may be introduced to the body leading to infection by means of a catheter, or during transplant surgery. It has displayed resistance to many forms of antibiotics, but at present remains treatable.

ACINETOBACTER SPP

This organism, which normally lives on the skin, can (usually in hospital settings) opportunistically become involved (per-haps after catheter use) in infections of the:

○ urinary tract
○ the lining of the brain – meningitis
○ and in peritonitis.

It has become widely resistant to antibiotics which previously controlled it.

MYCOBACTERIUM TUBERCULOSIS

Tuberculosis was until recently under control, at least in developed Western countries. However it has re-emerged as a major threat, and *Mycobacterium tuberculosis* can now be found in forms which are almost untreatable.

One of the major reasons for the development of resistance has been the tendency for some patients to fail to complete their courses of antibiotic treatment, one of the major factors that offers bacteria a chance to evolve defenses against a drug which is trying to kill them. It is as though a defending army were to show potential invaders how it proposed to defend itself and then decided to take a vacation, so allowing the invader time to work out new ways of overcoming it.

Among the most important background reasons for the emergence of multiple drug-resistant strains of *Mycobacterium tuberculosis* are thought to be:

○ failure of patients to complete courses of treatment – leading to mutant, resistant strains
○ deteriorating public health services due to economic constraints
○ poor training of health care workers in diagnosing and treating TB
○ delays in obtaining laboratory test results
○ use of only single-drug approaches to treat the infection (*see below*)
○ a dramatic increase in the numbers of susceptible people, often involving those who are impoverished and therefore malnourished, and/or homeless, and/or HIV positive and/or drug abusers
○ increasing migration into Western urban settings of people from areas where TB is endemic.

Many of these factors are beyond easy solution, and are political and economic in origin rather than medical. In other words, if everyone were well housed, well fed, well cared for and did not engage in practices which damage their immune systems, TB would vanish.

For successful care of TB today, there needs to be:

○ sound nutrition and hygiene
○ supervision which ensures that courses of antibiotic treatment are completed
○ the correct selection of a combination of antibiotic medications.

A treatment approach which involves using a combination of antibiotic drugs against the infection has been found to present the best option, since this offers multiple ways of killing or deactivating the invader.

When only single drugs are used, even if the course is followed through, *Mycobacterium tuberculosis* can respond with dramatically rapid genetic modifications in order to protect itself.

The number of cases in which treatment fails completely in dealing with TB is still relatively small, however when multiple drug-resistant tuberculosis (MDR-TB) does occur it is usually fatal, especially when this occurs in someone whose immune system is already compromised, for instance a person with an existing HIV infection or who is severely malnourished, such as a persistent drug abuser.

Sadly, hospital outbreaks of MDR-TB are increasing. Some of the reasons for this have been mentioned, but a summary is offered on pages 21–22 of other reasons why many bacteria have become immune to attack by antibiotics.

This is the cast – the good, the bad, and the frightening – we now need to become familiar with the way medicine tries to control them.

3: The Story So Far: A Brief History of Antibiotic Use

Before looking at antibiotics themselves, we should briefly examine antibacterial approaches, some of which are still in use, which preceded the discovery of antibiotics.

Before 1935 there were few successful medical methods for treating infections apart from procedures which went back hundreds of years, such as the use of an extract of cinchona bark for the treatment of malaria (from which quinine was eventually derived) and the use of ipecacuanha for some forms of dysentery.

During the early 20th century a few medications were developed in Germany for treatment of parasitic infections, but there were no antibacterial medications as such until the discovery of sulfur drugs, which were able to save lives in conditions which had previously been virtually untreatable.

The Sulfur Drugs

In 1935 it was announced that a drug had been developed, in Germany, of a sulfur derivative which could be used to treat commonly fatal streptococcal infections such as puerperal fever.

In the early 1930s over 1,000 young women were dying every year, in the UK, after childbirth because of infection of the bloodstream, from puerperal fever. Well over 100 out of every 100,000 births resulted in the mother becoming fatally infected in this way at this time.

When the new sulfonamide antibiotics were introduced in the mid-1930s, the figures for deaths from puerperal fever dropped dramatically, so that by 1940 the figure was down to around 20 deaths per 100,000 births. After the introduction of penicillin in the early 1940s, this figure dropped further so that there were fewer than 10 deaths per 100,000 births by 1950.

It was soon shown by research that the antibacterial effect of this drug resulted from the release from it, in the body, of a sulfur compound (sulfanilamide). This led to further research resulting in the production of sulfapyridine in 1938, which was capable of strong antibacterial effects against the microorganism responsible for pneumococcal pneumonia (*see Chapter 2*).

Research into sulfur drugs continued (and continues, although many scientists believe that drugs of this sort are no longer of much importance or usefulness). Professor Richard Lacey, writing in Geoffrey Cannons's comprehensive examination of the phenomenon of resistance, *Superbugs* (Virgin, 1995) says

> *Avoid all sulphonamides, except co-timoxazole in one special special situation – Pneumocystis carinii which is common in AIDS patients. [These drugs are] relatively toxic [many ill-effects]; obsolete. Better restricted for use in agriculture, as long as resultant meat and other human food contains no residues.*[1]

So what are the side-effects of sulfur drugs, which are still widely used?[2,3,4]

○ Formation of crystals can take place in the urine, which causes kidney blockage. This is said to be rare nowadays if the correct dosage is taken, but very serious if it does occur. Blood in the urine is an early sign.
○ A moderately severe fever and skin rash and damage to blood cells is an uncommon but possible hypersensitivity reaction.

○ Rarely, a severe reaction can occur in which a fever plus a skin rash also involves extensive ulceration of the mouth and/or the vagina. The eyes may become involved, leading commonly to blindness. This sometimes fatal condition is known as the Stevens-Johnson syndrome and usually relates to long-acting sulfur drugs, and is more common in young patients than adults. It is important to realize the degree of rarity of this sort of reaction – with an estimate of between 1 and 2 cases per 10 million doses prescribed.
○ Inflammation of the arteries can occur, as can inflammation of the heart muscle.
○ Damage to the bone marrow may occur, leading to several conditions – some serious – involving different blood cells, reduction in white blood cell levels, and various forms of anemia.
○ Liver damage may occur, as may lung diseases, but reports of these are extremely rare.

WHEN ARE SULFUR DRUGS NOW USED?

○ urinary tract infections – in combination with other drugs in treatment of *Pneumocystis carinii*, commonly in people with immune deficiency
○ sometimes in recurrent ear infections in children
○ previously widely used in meningitis and bacterial infections of the intestines, but less so now because of widespread resistance by the bacteria
○ for some sexually transmitted diseases such as chlamydia
○ sometimes in treating malaria and for some parasitic infections
○ in long-term control of conditions such as ulcerative colitis and Crohn's disease.

Much of the early research into antibiotics was diligent and painstaking, although some of the discoveries were almost accidental:

- Fleming's original revelation of the antibacterial effect of penicillin was a stroke of luck rather than genius. The spores of the mold from which the first penicillin was extracted had apparently floated out of one window (of a room where molds were being studied) in St. Mary's Hospital in London and onto culture dishes lying in Fleming's laboratory.

- Later another mold, now used for penicillin production (*Penicillium chrysogenum*), was discovered on a moldy melon (cantaloupe) found in a market in Peoria, Illinois.

- In 1953 an antibiotic (Helenine) which was used to treat some viral infections was isolated from *Penicillium funiculosum* after being noticed growing on the transparent (isinglass) cover of a photograph of the wife of the discoverer, a Dr Shope (his wife's name was Helen, hence the name given the antibiotic).

- Many antibiotics have been discovered in molds which live in the soil, where for millions of years microorganisms have competed with each other for nutrients and territory, and so have developed ways of attacking each other and of defending themselves. Not surprisingly, out of the tens of thousands of chemicals which these organisms produce to harm each other or defend themselves, some have been found which can be used in humans, to kill or damage other microorganisms which may be causing infection – without causing (too much) harm to the person being treated (though this is the hope rather than the reality, as we shall see).

- Cephalosporin antibiotics – such as the widely used antibiotics cefaclor and cefoxitin – were originally derived from microbes (molds) found in sewage.

- There are now literally tens of thousands of different antibiotic variations (*see Chapter 4 for a summary of the differences and details of some of the major versions*) and hundreds on the market, leading to great confusion in the minds of those who have to prescribe them. It is hard to know which (if any) is superior in many cases. Sometimes such decisions are easy and clear, but more often the doctor who has to prescribe has to make choices based on inadequate information. As Professor Garrod has stated,[5] 'A confident choice between them, for any given purpose, is one which few prescribers are qualified to make – indeed no one may be, since there is often no significant difference between the effects to be expected.'

O The laws of natural selection (and survival of the fittest) teach us that when assaulted by a toxic (to them) substance such as an antibiotic, some bacteria will survive, because they already have, or will develop, a natural immunity to the antibiotic. Those bacteria that survive will then be able to transmit this resistance to their descendants – this process lies at the heart of the superbug problem.

Antibiotics

Although there are a few records on the use of substances extracted from various molds to treat infection, going back thousands of years to ancient Egypt and indeed throughout recorded history, the modern era of antibiotic use dates back to around 1940.

PENICILLIN

Fleming had identified the antibiotic penicillin effect in 1929, however it was not until 1941 that extracts of the mold microbe *Penicillium notatum* were ready for use to treat infection. When enough of the first penicillin had been painstakingly gathered by the early researchers to treat patients, they were faced with the problem of too great a demand and too slow a production, especially after some of the initial cures, which were dramatic and newsworthy.

Conditions such as meningitis, septicemia and pneumonia became controllable for the first time, the early antibiotics proving superior in their effects to the sulfur drugs.

One early method of 'recycling' penicillin was to extract traces of it from the patient's urine and re-use it. After some years, methods of production improved and this recycling was stopped.

o Penicillin was initially used widely in childhood infections as well as for serious life-threatening infections in adults.
o Penicillin, and all antibiotics, are of no value whatever in treatment of viral illnesses, and yet in the early days through ignorance, and right up to the present, antibiotics were and are regularly prescribed for conditions not caused by bacteria at all.
o Allergic reactions to penicillin, as well as other types of reactions (usually mild and short-lived) including diarrhea and nausea, became (and remain) extremely common.
o One result of the enthusiastic and excessive use of penicillins was that by the late 1940s many disease-causing organisms had developed resistance to the early versions, and the energies of the pharmaceutical manufacturers were focused on the never-ending job of finding new variations which could control the resistant bacteria. In his prophetic book *When Antibiotics Fail*, Marc Lappe of the University of Illinois College of Medicine points out that over 23,000 different forms of penicillin had been developed during the period 1975 to 1986 (plus over 7,000 cephalosporins, 1,500 rifamycins, 3,000 tetracyclines, 750 lincomycins, 300 streptomycins and a further 1,000 aminoglycosides!).[6]

The painful truth is that the fortunes of many drug companies depend upon new resistances developing, new drugs appearing, and the cycle continuing forever. The problem for them is that it cannot, as options are increasingly limited in terms of new antibiotics. Other strategies will have to be found to deal with the super-resistance of the superbugs and the health crisis this is causing.

STREPTOMYCIN

By 1944 streptomycin had been developed (from the bacteria *Streptomycaes griseus*) – a breakthrough as this was able to treat tuberculosis effectively – for a while. It was not long, just a few years, before resistant strains appeared of *Mycobacterium tuberculosis*.

Streptomycin was also soon found to be extremely toxic and is in decline in usefulness in Western industrialized countries, although in many under-developed countries it is widely and inappropriately used (along with other antibiotics) – often without the need for prescription – causing a potential disease time-bomb in often malnourished populations.

According to the British Medical Association,

> These potent drugs are effective against a broad range of bacteria, but they are not as widely used as some other antibiotics because they have to be given by injection, and they also have potentially serious side-effects.[7]

Their use is therefore limited to hospital treatment of serious infections.

Possible adverse effects include:

○ damage to the nerves of the ear
○ damage to the kidneys
○ severe skin rashes.

Over the more than 50 years since penicillin and streptomycin appeared, a host of new antibiotics have emerged and continue to reach the market every year.

CHLORAMPHENICOL

In the late 1940s came the chloramphenicol drugs, a 'broad-spectrum' antibiotic which was apparently effective against many different microorganisms. These drugs were originally widely and enthusiastically used to treat everything from gonorrhea to blood infections and gastroenteritis.

Unfortunately however for the manufacturers of chloramphenicol, some extremely serious side-effects soon began to appear – albeit in only a small number of patients – including potentially fatal aplastic anemia. It also caused major problems when used to treat young children, and so chloramphenicol's use in industrialized nations has now diminished to very special situations only, such as:

○ typhoid fever (which means that it is still widely used in underdeveloped countries where typhoid is widespread)
○ some forms of meningitis
○ life-threatening chest infections
○ where nothing else is working to control a serious bacterial infection, so that there is little to lose by trying something as potentially dangerous as a form of chloramphenicol.

The irony here is that because chloramphenicol antibiotics are now used so rarely, bacterial resistance has not been developing against them as rapidly, making these highly toxic drugs possible choices if superinfection occurs. This leads to the thought that if the bug doesn't get you, the treatment just might.

TETRACYCLINES

In the late 1940s, new antibiotics derived from soil microorganisms appeared. These have an even wider target range than the chloramphenicol drugs – and are known as tetracyclines. One of the most popular of the tetracyclines first appeared in 1950 – oxytetracycline, which is still very much in use.

These antibiotics were and are used to treat infections of many sorts, including those of the eyes, ears, throat, digestive and urinary tracts, acne and a number of sexually transmitted diseases. Unfortunately, as with many other antibiotics, tetracyclines are also widely used in agriculture and have entered the food chain.

The excessive and indiscriminate use of these extremely broad-spectrum antibiotics has resulted in bacterial resistance appearing which limits their use – though, given their side-effects, some might consider this a blessing.

Side-effects to tetracycline drugs are numerous according to the British Medical Association, which summarizes them thus:

> A major drawback to the use of tetracycline antibiotics in young children and pregnant women is that they can discolour developing teeth. When given by mouth they have to be administered in high doses to reach effective levels in the blood (because they are poorly absorbed through the intestines). Such high doses increase the likelihood of diarrhoea.

Short-term reactions include:

○ allergic reactions
○ sore and itchy rectum
○ sore tongue
○ swallowing difficulties.

Long-term problems relate to the demolition job that tetracyclines do on the bowel flora, the friendly bacteria which detoxify our intestines and manufacture B-vitamins for us, and above all which keep yeasts under control.

When tetracycline drugs are used, often for months on end to treat acne, for example, an overgrowth of yeast in the bowel is almost certain, and it can take years to put this right. (*See Chapters 7 and 8 for details of aspects of these effects and what you can do about them, as well as Chapter 9 for probiotic strategies to help reverse this damage.)*

CEPHALOSPORINS

As mentioned above, the cephalosporins (such as cefaclor) were first extracted from fungal spores found in sewage in the mid-1940s. They were initially fairly toxic, but with steady development of more refined versions they have become less so.

Cephalosporins act in similar ways to penicillin-type drugs, have a wide spectrum and are fairly well tolerated. Their use is mainly in treatment of infections of the chest, urinary tract, liver and gall bladder, as well as for gonorrhea. They are commonly being used prophylactically, before surgery for example, and are frequently used when penicillin antibiotics fail to control infection. They can be administered either by mouth or by injection.

Side-effects include:

○ allergy – relatively common – in up to 10 percent of patients, in the form of rashes, fever and sickness
○ severe blood clotting problems – relatively rare.

Resistance is gradually building to many of the major drugs in this group, in a number of important disease-causing microbes, including *Staphylococcas aureus*, *Klebsiella*, *E. coli* and *Pseudomonas aeruginosa*.

THE MACROLIDE, GLYCOPEPTIDES AND LINCOSAMIDE DRUGS

In the early 1950s, drugs in the class of broad-spectrum antibiotics known as macrolides appeared. The most notable of these, and the only one still in major use, is erythromycin.

Erythromycin is used as an alternative to penicillin and cephalosporin drugs and has a particular usefulness in the treatment of Legionnaires' disease (a rare form of pneumonia). It carries risks relating to liver damage and so is used cautiously.

The glycopeptide drugs include the toxic, expensive and hence very rarely used vancomycin. Its potency against super-bugs such as *S. aureus* (*see Chapter 2*) makes this a drug held in reserve, and because of this resistance to it is low. Once again we see the irony of the savior drug being so toxic that it carries dangers all its own.

Among the side-effects of vancomycin are:

○ a bright red flushing (combined with severe itching) of all or part of the body ('red-man' reaction)
○ swelling of the mucous membranes
○ cardiovascular collapse (rare)
○ damage to the ears possibly leading to irreversible deafness
○ damage to the kidneys
○ serious blood diseases involving the white blood cells.

But remember – it could save your life at the same time.

The lincosamide drugs such as lincomycin appeared in the early 1960s, and are used mainly for treatment of extremely serious infections of bones, joints and the abdomen which fail to respond to other antibiotics. They too are therefore 'kept in reserve' because of their side-effects.

As the British Medical Association explains, 'they are more likely to cause serious disruption of bacterial activity in the bowel than other antibiotics.' This highlights the vital importance of maintaining the health of the friendly bacteria, and since all antibiotics damage these it is safe to assume that the lincosamide antibiotics are absolutely devastating.

Quinolone Drugs

These represent a more recent antibacterial development (1970s onwards) and a terrifying prospect.

Over the past 30 years or so frantic research work has continued to keep up with the resistance patterns in infectious bacteria, and only a few novel antibiotics have appeared, all others having been new versions of old models. It has therefore become clearer to researchers that the future does not lie in reworking old ideas, as this vein was virtually worked out.

So it was back to the drawing board in order to investigate synthetic options, no longer relying on modifications of Nature's natural products.

Out of this research came a group of antibacterial drugs, acting as antibiotics but not derived from living organisms – the quinolones (and their cousins, the fluoroquinolones) including nalidixic acid, pipemedic acid, cinoxacin and difloxacin.

Early versions of these drugs have been withdrawn because of, it is said, 'increasing resistance and the relative frequency of central nervous system side-effects.'

Current versions, which are mainly used to treat urinary tract infections, are said to produce infrequent side-effects including the usual diarrhea, allergic reactions, skin rashes and fever.

Geoffrey Cannon, however, cautions in his book *Superbugs* that this is potentially only the tip of the iceberg. Among his reasons for this are:

○ The mode of action of these drugs is to alter the genetic material of the bacteria being attacked, and there remains a chance (denied by scientists) that this could also modify the genetic material of the host – you.
○ Enormous quantities are being used in agriculture, most notably in fish farming, and tens of thousands of kilos of the drugs are entering the ecosystems via rivers and the sea, with totally unpredictable effects long term.

○ Some of the drug leaves the human body via urine and enters the waste disposal and water recycling systems of the area. Some of this inevitably finds its way back into drinking water – with what long-term effects?

○ Because these drugs are effective against the disease-causing bacteria they are targeting (until resistance is acquired) but are not at all harmful to the friendly bacteria, this offers the chance for our normal flora, such as *L. acidophilus*, to mutate into harmful forms. This has already happened, according to Cannon.[8]

There is no doubt whatever that antibiotics have saved millions of lives, and continue to do so. There is also no doubt that antibiotics have been (and are being) misused, and we are seeing the signs of the horrors this will produce: untreatable superinfections.

Dr. Joseph Pizzorno, President of Bastyr University, Seattle, states,

> *While antibiotics are very useful when the body's immune system is overwhelmed, their excessive use (both medically and in agriculture) causes many problems. Overuse can damage the immune system, cause overgrowth of Candida fungus [see Chapter 7] in the intestines and vagina, and spur the development of antibiotic-resistant bacteria that can evade the immune system ... it is increasingly difficult to find antibiotics that are effective against pneumococcal infections of the ear, respiratory tract, staphylococcal infections of the skin, and gonococcal infections of the genitals.[9]*

As time passes, so research uncovers more and more variations on the theme of controlling infection by bacteria, and as time passes so do the bacteria under attack develop ways of altering their own characteristics, so that they become immune to the onslaught.

This is the never-ending game of 'catch-up' which the pharmaceutical industry has to play if it is to maintain its ability to control or kill infectious microorganisms. Unfortunately, as indicated in the previous chapter, the bacteria seem to be winning at the moment.

In their natural environment bacteria have learned to deal with chemicals (for example the natural antibiotics produced by their fungal and mold enemies who compete with them for food and space) in many ways. For example, bacteria learn to produce an enzyme which inactivates part of the antibiotic; others, increasingly, have modified their structure so that they have fewer parts (attachment sites) on their surface to which the antibiotic can latch on and do its job.

Other changes which have taken place include a frightening prospect in which bacteria have learned to live *without cell walls*. This makes them similar to the stealth bomber which is invisible to radar. They have become 'stealth bacteria', invisible to the defense systems of the body which depend upon being able to recognize enemies by means of the chemicals (proteins) on their surface. What if there is no surface?

There is no doubt that the high hopes of the early work in antibiotics are fading.

The late Professor L. Garrod, in his contribution to a chapter by Professor David Greenwood of Queens Medical Centre, Nottingham, England, in a major textbook on antibiotics and chemotherapy, has stated,

> *Not only is the action of any new [antibiotic] drug on an individual bacteria still unpredictable on a theoretical basis, but so are its effects on the body itself. Most of the toxic effects of antibiotics have come to light only after extensive use, and even now no one can explain their affinity for some of the organs attacked.*

He continues,

> *Some of the [antibiotic] drugs which it is necessary to use are far from ideal, whether because of toxicity or of unsatisfactory properties ... moreover, microbic resistance is a constant threat to the future usefulness of almost any [antibiotic] drug. It seems unlikely that any totally new antibiotic remains to be discovered, since those of recent origin have similar properties to others already known. It therefore will be wise to husband our resources, and employ them in such a way as to preserve them.*[10]

This is the message which this book is promoting, that antibiotics as we know them are useful in life-threatening situations only, and that if we wish to maintain that chance of a life-saving potential, we need to stop using them in the way they are being used today.

The Future?

Medical science suggests that to be an effective antibiotic a substance must have certain characteristics:

○ It must either kill or inhibit microbes.
○ It must be able to be used in the human body without causing severe undesirable side-effects. We will examine some additional short- and long-term side-effects in Chapters 7 and 8 – you can then decide for yourself whether this criterion is being met!
○ If at all possible the antibiotic should be stable, soluble, and be only slowly excreted by the body.

How is medical science dealing with these demands in the face of increasing bacterial resistance? A number of approaches are being studied to overcome these problems:

○ Old drugs are being modified to make them more soluble, more stable, more long-lasting in the body, less toxic, and if at all possible with greater antimicrobial potency.
○ New antibiotics are being developed, but few have more than a marginal benefit when compared with those already available.
○ Genetic modification is being attempted to make bacteria more vulnerable to the antibiotics currently available.
○ Combinations of antibiotics, or much more potent antibiotics (with more side-effects) are being used in certain cases to ensure success in controlling certain microbes. However if such strategies are overused, resistance will develop to these methods as well. There are a variety of tactics whereby antibiotics can be used in combination or in particular ways so that the resistance factor can be reduced – it can never, however, be totally eliminated.

Alternatives

Other choices exist – an examination of other (than antibiotic) ways of inhibiting infection as well as methods for immune enhancement. These will all be looked at later in the book.

Based on the evidence touched on in this chapter, it is suggested that antibiotics should be kept in reserve for essential use only – where life is under threat.

Other ways should be learned and adopted which can encourage the natural defenses of the body (the immune system) to do one of the key jobs they were designed for, the control of invading bacteria. Chapters 5 and 6 will highlight many immune-enhancing methods. However now we will look at precisely how antibiotics work.

4: How the Major Antibiotics Work – and Some Problems[1,2,3,4,5]

One definition of an antibiotic is that it is a substance derived from a living organism which enters the body, either by mouth or injection, and which then travels via the bloodstream to reach an infected area where it either kills, or in some other way deactivates, an invading microorganism.

This definition means that the antibiotic acts 'systemically' and not just locally.[6]

Another definition which is widely accepted is that an antibiotic is a substance produced by microorganisms which is antagonistic to the growth or life of other microorganisms when highly diluted.

The words 'when highly diluted' are important in this definition. They help to make clear that antibiotics are not substances like the ones produced by animals and humans which inhibit bacteria when at full strength, for example digestive acids which, as part of their role in digesting food, also help to control bacterial activity in the stomach by maintaining acidity at the appropriate level to achieve this.

A substance which is placed onto the surface of the body to control bacterial infection is known as an *antiseptic* rather than an *antibiotic*.

Synthetic substances (which are not derived from living organisms) that deactivate or kill bacteria are not antibiotics but are called simply 'antibacterial' drugs.

The sulfur drugs and the newer quinolone drugs, described in Chapter 3, are therefore antibacterial and not antibiotic, although in many cases they perform much the same task, of controlling bacterial infection.

All true antibiotics now being used to treat infection are products of microorganisms, although many have been artificially modified by science to alter the ways in which they function, and some are now manufactured synthetically.

How Do They Work?

Antibiotics (and antibacterial drugs) can have two distinct and different ways of doing their work:

1 If they are *bactericidal* they actually kill bacteria.
2 If they are *bacteriostatic* they interfere with the way in which the bacteria reproduce themselves or function, and so, by one means or another, slow down or stop bacterial activity without actually killing the bacteria. As we will see later in this chapter, there are a number of ways in which antibiotics can achieve the task of damaging and inhibiting bacteria.

Bacteria are all around us, in the air, on almost everything we touch, by the billion on our skin, in our mouth, ears, nose and eyes, and by the trillions in our digestive tract, where over 400 different species – most of them friendly and useful – live.

We have lived with bacteria since humans have existed, and indeed according to evolutionary theory we are ourselves – along with most life on earth – descendants of the original life-forms, bacteria.

As we will see in more detail in Chapter 7, we depend upon the symbiotic relationship which exists between bacteria and ourselves for life itself. Unfortunately the methods involved in treating infection by means of antibiotics neglect to take adequate account of the devastation which these drugs cause to the essential bacterial colonies living in and on us.

Antibiotics do their work by either killing or, more usually, by interfering with one or other aspect of the physiology of the bacteria they are targeting, so deactivating them.

As we have seen in Chapter 2, bacteria are not uniform; they have different features. Some live in an oxygen-rich environment, others are happier without oxygen, and some can adapt to both environments.

They have many other individual characteristics, and different antibiotics have been devised which can exploit these bacterial differences and unique characteristics in order to deactivate or eliminate them. For example, as discussed in Chapter 2, in general (there are exceptions) some bacteria are gram-positive (they stain blue/purple when tested) while others are gram-negative (they stain pink/red when tested). This ability to be stained one way or the other classifies the bacteria and helps in the decision as to which type of antibiotic to use in trying to control it. This is because some antibiotics will only work on gram-negative bacteria and other antibiotics only work on gram-positive ones.

Therefore there is no universally effective antibiotic; each drug 'works' to control some but not other hostile bacteria – while at the same time causing harm to some but not other of the friendly bacteria.

Antibiotics can be said to work by 'selective toxicity', in which they take advantage of differences between the way a particular bacteria is constructed or functions as compared with the way the cells of the tissues being infected (yours and mine) are constructed and function.

Some antibiotics devastate the intestinal flora, while others have a lesser effect, and no antibiotics actually enhance the normal flora. It is only the degree of harm they cause to the flora that varies.

ANTIBIOTICS AND THE IMMUNE SYSTEM

Some antibiotics are claimed actually to improve immune function, either by weakening and making more vulnerable the bacteria being targeted, or by actually increasing the activity of the immune cells which are doing the attacking. The majority of antibiotics have neither effect, simply doing the attacking of the bacteria, in one way or another (*see below*).

Other antibiotics actually weaken the way the immune system responds to bacterial infection (including tetracycline and erythromycin, which are discussed later in this chapter).[7]

Different Types of Antibacterials and Antibiotics and Their Main Properties

THE SULFA (SULFONAMIDE) ANTIBACTERIAL DRUGS

Commonly used sulfonamides include Cotrimoxazole and Sulfacetamide.

O The sulfa antibacterial drugs were developed before antibiotics, and are still in limited use.
O Unlike antibiotics, these drugs are not derived from living microorganisms, but are chemicals.
O They were first developed from a deep red dye called prontosil which is turned into sulfonamide inside the body.
O They interfere with the way bacteria manufacture an essential nutrient needed to survive, folic acid. They do this by stopping the release of an enzyme which is needed by the bacteria to manufacture folic acid.
O Without the folic acid the bacteria die.
O Bacteria have, to a very large extent, become resistant to sulfonamide and the sulfa drugs.
O Supporters believe that the sulfa drugs are still particularly useful in urinary tract infections.

- Other areas of usefulness are said to include chlamydial pneumonia and certain middle ear infections, as well as in a number of preparations for use on the skin, in the eyes and on the outer ears.
- Treatment of leprosy has been effective, over a period of several years of therapy, using a drug which is related to the sulfonamides, dapsone, although the organism responsible is now becoming resistant to it.
- Common but not serious side-effects include loss of appetite, skin rashes, feelings of extreme drowsiness and nausea, as well as allergic reactions.
- Rare but serious side-effects (danger is reduced by avoiding long courses of treatment with these drugs) include:
  - development of crystals in the kidneys (made less likely by consumption of high levels of fluid during treatment with these drugs)
  - liver damage – can be severe, and so the drugs are avoided if liver function is already damaged
  - bone marrow damage – possibly leading to lowered levels of protective white blood cells and increased likelihood of infection.

An example of the uses, cautions, and side-effects of one of the sulfa antibacterial drugs – **Cotrimoxazole**, which is mainly a sulfa drug with a small element of another antibacterial drug, trimethoprim.[8]

- *Main indications:* respiratory and gastrointestinal infections; infections of the skin and ears
- *Specific uses:* treating prostatitis, gonorrhea, pneumocystis pneumonia
- *Not normally prescribed for:* pregnant women, breastfeeding women, infants under six weeks, people over 60 (side-effects are more likely)

○ *Dosage and duration of treatment:* by injection, tablet or liquid; usually for five days, taken twice daily. The medication should not be stopped before the end of the course or recurrence is likely.
○ *Special instructions:* drink plenty of fluids.
○ *Main common side-effects:* nausea, vomiting, rash and itching
○ *Main uncommon side-effects:* diarrhea, sore tongue, headache and jaundice, drowsiness, loss of appetite and allergic reactions
○ *Long-term use* can lead to folic acid deficiency and blood abnormalities.
○ *Contraindications:* Anyone who has liver or kidney problems, a blood disorder, or who is allergic to sulfonamide drugs, suffers from porphyria or is taking other medications requires special consideration as to whether Cotrimoxazole is suitable.

PENICILLINS

Commonly used penicillins include amoxycillin, ampicillin, benzylpenicillin.

○ Penicillins were the first antibiotic drugs.
○ The penicillins (just like the cephalosporins, which are discussed below) kill a wide range of bacteria and are therefore said to be bactericidal; many are 'broad-spectrum', able to kill many different bacterial strains in the treatment of many conditions involving almost all organs and systems of the body, with particularly wide applications in ear, nose, throat, respiratory, bone and joint, genital tract as well as kidney and urinary tract infections.
○ They (like the cephalosporins) are able to act on bacteria which are sensitive to them by interfering with the chemicals involved in the normal formation of the bacteria's cell walls, causing the bacteria to disintegrate without doing the same to the human cells they come in contact with.

O Some penicillin drugs are useful taken by mouth, while others need to be injected.

O Penicillin drugs are eliminated from the body in the urine.

O They are relatively non-toxic to humans, however allergic reactions are common and these are very occasionally severe – even fatal.

O Diarrhea is the commonest symptom noted when these drugs are administered, largely because of damage caused to the friendly flora in the bowel – see Chapters 9 and 10 for strategies to help reduce this danger.

O Because some penicillins have a broad spectrum of activity they have been known to cause what is known as super-infection, in which there is an explosion of activity of opportunistic bacteria, fungi or yeasts after the antibiotic has dealt with (in this case killed) the original infecting bacteria.

O Because of widespread use in farming, traces of these drugs are found in meat and dairy products. People who consume the resulting food products therefore offer a chance for bacteria living inside them to become resistant to antibiotic treatment.

O Bacterial resistance to most penicillin antibiotics is now widespread, with some strains of bacteria (e.g. most staphylococci) having become completely resistant. The bacterial resistance is achieved mainly by the bacteria 'learning' how to produce enzymes which can neutralize the ability of the antibiotic to affect them.

O Bacteria can also modify their structure to reduce the sites which the antibiotics can attack.

O Newer penicillins have been devised to overcome these resistance tactics, for example the co-amoxiclav drug azlocillin. In time, with sufficient use, these too will help to produce resistant strains of the bacteria they are trying to kill. The cycle of 'improved' drug leading to greater resistance leading to yet more improved versions of the drug will continue until the folly of this approach becomes absolutely obvious, and focus switches to enhancing immune function rather than trying to find bigger and better drugs to control the organisms which are taking advantage of conditions suitable for their activities.

An example of the uses, cautions, and side-effects of one of the penicillin antibiotic drugs – **amoxycillin**.[9]

○ *Main indications:* ear, nose and throat infections, respiratory tract infections, cystitis, 'simple' gonorrhea and some skin infections
○ *Not normally prescribed for:* infants and children, unless at reduced dosage
○ *Dosage and duration of treatment:* varies; will be individually prescribed by the doctor. It is usually taken via sachet, tablets, capsules, liquid or injection, three times daily. The medication should not be stopped before the end of the course or recurrence is likely, and would in any case encourage the evolution of resistant strains.
○ *Main common side-effect:* a rash, which does not necessarily indicate an allergy
○ *Main uncommon side-effects:* an allergic reaction which includes fever, swelling of mouth and tongue, itching and breathing problems
○ *Long-term use* is unusual; short courses are the norm.
○ *Contraindications:* anyone taking oral contraceptives may develop breakthrough bleeding and the contraceptive effect may be reduced.
○ *Special cautions:* anyone with kidney problems, allergy history (asthma, hayfever), previous antibiotic allergy, ulcerative colitis, glandular fever or those taking other medications, will require special consideration as to whether the use of amoxycillin is suitable.

CEPHALOSPORINS

Commonly used cephalosporins include cefaclor, cefoxitin.

○ Cephalosporins (which are very similar to penicillins) kill a wide range of bacteria and are therefore said to be bactericidal; many are 'broad-spectrum', able to kill many different bacterial strains in the treatment of many conditions involving almost all organs and systems of the body, with particularly wide applications in ear, nose, throat, respiratory, bone and joint, genital tract as well as kidney and urinary tract infections.

○ They are particularly useful in serious infections of the urinary tract because they become concentrated in the kidneys before excretion.

○ Just like the penicillins, the cephalosporins are able to act on bacteria which are sensitive to them by interfering with the chemicals involved in the normal formation of the bacteria's cell walls, causing the bacteria to disintegrate without doing the same to the human cells they contact.

○ The cephalosporins are often used when penicillins fail to control an infection.

○ They are used particularly to control the staphylococci, streptococci and some gram-negative bacteria such as the coliforms.

○ Some cephalosporins can be taken by mouth, but many are given by injection.

○ They have evolved over the years, and newer versions are relatively non-toxic to humans with a wide range of use, with particular emphasis on gall bladder and urinary tract infections as well as use before surgery to prevent infection.

○ Resistance to earlier versions has become widespread, but currently used cephalosporins are relatively capable of overcoming bacterial defenses which have developed over the years.

○ They are relatively non-toxic to humans, however allergic reactions are common and these are very occasionally severe – even fatal. Anyone who has already had an allergic reaction to a penicillin drug should not be given a cephalosporin medication, as the chance of a reaction is high.

○ Anyone with kidney problems should be extremely cautious regarding cephalosporin medication.

○ Diarrhea is the commonest symptom noted when these drugs are administered, largely because of damage caused to the friendly flora in the bowel – see Chapters 9 and 10 for strategies to help reduce this danger.

○ Nausea and vomiting may accompany diarrhea as side-effects, but are usually mild.

○ A potentially serious (but relatively rare) side-effect of these drugs involves interference with normal blood clotting which can result in excessive bleeding. This happens more frequently in the elderly.

○ Because most cephalosporins have a broad spectrum of activity they have been known to cause what is known as superinfection, in which there is an explosion of activity of opportunistic bacteria, fungi or yeasts after the antibiotic has dealt with (in this case killed) the original infecting bacteria.

○ Professor Marc Lappe reports that when cephalosporins are used to treat infections in women they result in damage to the normal flora of the vagina. 'The devastation of the natural residents leads to overgrowth of E. coli, Pseudomonas as well as disease causing Bacteroides.'

An example of the uses, cautions, and side-effects of one of the cephalosporin antibiotic drugs – **cefaclor**.[10]

○ *Main indications:* infections of the respiratory tract, sinuses, skin, urinary tract and the middle ear. It is commonly effective against some bacteria which are resistant to penicillin drugs.

○ *Not normally prescribed for:* breastfeeding women as the drug passes through the milk to the baby; infants and children require a reduced dosage

○ *Dosage and duration of treatment:* usually only short courses are prescribed. The antibiotic is taken orally in the form of sustained-release tablets, capsules, or liquid, taken three times daily. The medication should not be stopped before the end of the course or recurrence is likely, and also as this may encourage the evolution of resistant strains (those that survive the medication because it is stopped too soon may 'learn' to defend against it another time).

○ *Main common side-effect:* diarrhea, which is usually not severe but should alert you to the fact that the normal bowel flora are being damaged, calling for the sort of strategy detailed in Chapter 9

○ *Main less common side-effects:* usually considered to be the result of allergy, include nausea and vomiting, itching, skin rash, fever, and swollen and painful joints

○ *Contraindications:* anyone with kidney problems, previous antibiotic allergy, a history of bleeding disorders or who is taking other medications will require special consideration as to whether the use of cefaclor is suitable.

AMINOGLYCOSIDES

Commonly used aminoglycosides include neomycin, streptomycin, gentamycin.

○ The aminoglycosides were the next major antibiotic group developed after the penicillins.

○ Along with the cephalosporins, the aminoglycoside drugs are probably the most expensive antibiotics ever produced.

○ These are fairly toxic, broad-spectrum, bactericidal antibiotics which are active against gram-negative bacteria.

○ The aminoglycosides are active against some of the most potent disease-causing bacteria (unless the bacteria have acquired resistance), including *Staphylococcus aureus, Mycobacterium tuberculosis.*

○ The aminoglycosides tend to be prescribed less frequently than some other forms of antibiotic because they usually have to be administered by intramuscular injection and because of the possibility of side-effects.

○ Their use is largely confined to serious bacterial infection – for example streptomycin is sometimes used for treatment of tuberculosis or bubonic plague – and they are usually prescribed along with other antibiotics.

○ Spectinomycin is used for those forms of gonorrhea which have become resistant to penicillin – medical protocols recommend that both partners should be treated, with women receiving twice the dosage prescribed for men.

○ Neomycin is often prescribed orally for some forms of liver failure and before surgery on the digestive tract because it so effectively destroys the flora of the bowel.

○ The aminoglycosides are used to a greater extent in hospital settings rather than as general prescription antibiotics, except for some applications, such as neomycin for skin application, or in the form of nose, ear or eye drops.

○ Aminoglycosides achieve their effect by preventing the bacteria they are attacking from synthesizing protein, so preventing them from reproducing themselves.

○ They are not absorbed in the digestive tract (which is why they are usually given by injection) and so aminoglycoside drugs are sometimes prescribed to be taken by mouth for digestive and urinary tract infections.

○ Damage to the bowel flora is widespread when such drugs are used – lincomycin, neomycin and kanamycin cause so much damage that Candida and *Staphylococcus aureus* overgrowth is not uncommon. Resistance to these drugs by bacteria is widespread and growing, although where the use of the aminoglycosides has been reduced, resistance has also dropped.

○ Different bacterial species are often able to transfer resistance to each other once it has been acquired (known as 'cross-resistance').

○ Pregnant women and people with kidney problems should not be prescribed a number of the aminoglycosides, for example streptomycin.

○ Among the side-effects noted with the aminoglycosides are:

○ if given by injection, pain and irritation at the puncture site is common.

○ local nerves may also become irritated and inflamed, leading to neuritis.

○ hearing difficulties, including irreversible deafness, usually only if dosage is high and more likely in older patients

○ kidney failure, especially in elderly patients (rare but serious)

○ aplastic anemia (rare but very serious)

○ high temperature

○ severe skin rashes and itching occurs in about one patient in 20 receiving these drugs.

○ dizziness and headaches (common)

○ numbness around the mouth (common).

An example of the uses, cautions, and side-effects of one of the aminoglycoside antibiotic drugs – **gentamycin**.[11]

○ *Specific uses:* treating serious and complicated infections in hospital settings involving the lungs, bones, joints, wounds, urinary tract infections, and conditions such as septicemia (blood infection), peritonitis, and meningitis. It is also used as a cream, ointment, or drops for eye and ear infections. It is used in combination with penicillin to treat (or prevent) heart valve infections (endocarditis).

○ *Not normally prescribed for:* the creams and drops represent no risk for pregnant women, but injections are avoided for pregnant or breastfeeding women. Infants require reduced dosages, and people over 60 are regarded as being at risk from side-effects and so reduced dosages are used.

○ *Dosage and duration of treatment:* by injection, not usually for longer than 10 days due to the risk of kidney damage. Injections are usually given every eight hours, while eye ointments are suggested every 6 to 12 hours and ear drops every 4 to 8 hours. The medication should not be stopped before the end of the course or recurrence is likely, and also as this may encourage the evolution of resistant strains (survivors may 'learn' to defend against it another time).

○ *Main common side-effects:* none

○ *Uncommon side-effects:* nausea and vomiting, dizziness, skin rashes with itching, ringing in the ears (tinnitus), loss of hearing, blood in the urine, headaches, and numbness. Combined with drugs such as vancomycin (used to treat resistant infections with superbugs) the potential for side-effects such as deafness and kidney disease will be increased.

○ *Long-term use:* may lead to severe kidney disease and hearing problems.

○ *Contraindications:* anyone with kidney problems, hearing difficulties, previous allergy to aminoglycoside antibiotics, or those taking other medications will require special consideration as to whether the use of gentamycin is suitable.

TETRACYCLINES

Commonly used tetracyclines include tetracycline, oxytetracycline and doxycycline.

○ The tetracyclines were discovered in 1948 and are broad-spectrum bacteriostatic antibiotics which were widely used in the treatment of a large number of infectious conditions ranging from pneumonia to bladder infections, conjunctivitis to cholera.
○ They are also active against protozoa (spirochete parasites) – such as the organism which causes Lyme disease and is carried by ticks.
○ Because of the wide range of bacterial resistance which developed to the tetracyclines, they are currently being used far less (in some countries) than in the past, and where this has happened, in the UK for example, resistance has also decreased as a result.
○ They are usually taken orally in liquid, capsule or tablet form.
○ The conditions for which they are now most usually prescribed are:

  ○ pneumonia which is due to chlamydia, rickettsia, or mycoplasma
  ○ urethritis and pelvic inflammatory disease due to chlamydia
  ○ Lyme disease
  ○ brucellosis
  ○ chronic bronchitis.

○ The action of the tetracyclines is similar to that of the aminoglycosides: they prevent the normal synthesis of protein by the bacteria which they are attacking, so preventing the bacteria from reproducing or surviving.

○ The use of tetracyclines in farming is enormous – both in meat production, where they are used to promote growth (beef, pigs, chickens), and in fruit production to increase the growth rate of trees. The impact of this on human health is unpredictable but probably enormous.

○ Among the common and less common side-effects are:

   ○ a tendency to stain teeth a mottled yellow/brown
   ○ nausea, vomiting, and diarrhea – which shows the likelihood there is for these drugs to damage the normal flora of the bowels
   ○ extreme irritation of the lining of the intestines can also occur with tetracycline drugs, leading to pseudo-membranous colitis, a severe and potentially serious bleeding of the bowel.
   ○ superinfection is possible, resulting from the destruction of specific target bacteria and the chance this gives to other bacteria to take advantage of the situation. This can involve many different organisms including Candida, *Staphylococcus aureus*, *Proteus* and others.
   ○ yeast overgrowth (superinfection) of the intestines – Candida – which occurs when the normal bowel flora are damaged. See Chapters 7 and particularly 9 and 10 for more information and for strategies to reduce this likelihood.
   ○ a sensitivity to light (photophobia) – this symptom is not common and is more likely if the tetracycline drug demeclocycline is used.
   ○ bone deformity if bones are still growing – the tetracycline drugs are not usually prescribed for children under 12.
   ○ aggravation of existing kidney problems is possible and serious.
   ○ skin problems often occur because of changes in the local fatty acid status of the skin, involving increased

amounts of particular oils (triglycerides) and the destruction of the normal, harmless skin bacteria *Propionibacterium acnes* – which allows undesirable bacteria such as *Staphylococcus aureus* to colonize the skin, which can result in boils.

○ Professor Marc Lappe reports that in 1977 researchers found that tetracycline (and chloramphenicol) both depressed immune function to a great extent, so reducing the chance of a defense against invading bacteria being effective. This is confirmed by Dr Curtis Gemmel of Glasgow's Royal Infirmary and Head of the Department of Bacteriology at Glasgow Medical School, who says that tetracycline exerts its ability to depress immune function by removing calcium and magnesium from immune cells such as the phagocytes which 'eat' invading bacteria, thereby weakening them (*see Chapter 5 for more detail on the immune system*).[12]

○ Resistance to the tetracyclines is widespread but is not yet a major problem in treating those conditions where the tetracyclines are a first-choice antibiotic – however, *Staphylococcus aureus* is now largely resistant to tetracycline, as are *Salmonella* species and most entero-bacteria.

An example of the uses, cautions, and side-effects of one of the tetracycline antibiotic drugs – **doxycycline**.[13]

○ *Main indications:* respiratory and urinary tract infections as well as infections of the eyes, skin, prostate and gastrointestinal tracts
○ *Specific uses:* treating chlamydia infections and acne
○ *Not normally prescribed for:* pregnant women, breastfeeding women (it turns teeth yellow/brown) or anyone under the age of 12 for the same reasons, as well as for effects on growing bones

---

○ *Dosage and duration of treatment:* the medication is taken orally as tablets or capsules and the duration of treatment will be decided by the doctor based on the particular situation. The medication should not be stopped before the end of the course, or recurrence is likely, and also as this may encourage the evolution of resistant strains (those that survive the medication because it is stopped too soon may 'learn' to defend against it another time).

○ *Special instructions:* avoid milk when taking this drug.

○ *Main common side-effects:* nausea and indigestion which can be reduced by taking the antibiotic at meal times

○ *Main uncommon side-effects:* diarrhea, skin rash and itching, skin sensitivity to light (a rash appears)

○ *Long-term use* is not thought to cause problems.

○ *Contraindications:* anyone with liver problems, previous allergy to tetracycline antibiotics, or who is taking other medications will require special consideration as to whether the use of doxycycline is suitable.

LINCOSAMIDES

There are just two lincosamide antibiotics – lincomycin and clindamycin.

○ As with many antibiotics, the lincosamides were first extracted from soil bacteria.

○ The lincosamides are not commonly used because medical science recognizes just how severe a degree of damage they cause to the bowel flora.

○ The lincosamides work by preventing the normal synthesis of protein by the bacteria which they are attacking, so preventing it from reproducing or surviving.

○ The main use of the lincosamides is in:

○ treatment of bone, joint and abdominal infections (such as peritonitis)

- female genital infections (usually when other antibiotics have failed), or for
- people who are allergic to penicillin or cephalosporins.
- They are active only against gram-positive bacteria as well as some mycoplasmas and protozoas (*see Chapter 3 for more information*).
- They quite commonly cause severe diarrhea as a side-effect. This can lead to *Pseudomembranous colitis*, which involves bowel bleeding. This is more likely in people over 60, and may persist long after the antibiotic use is finished.
- Resistance has been shown in the staphylococci to the lincosamide drugs (lincomycin is not much used, having been largely replaced by clindamycin).

An example of the uses, cautions, and side-effects of one of the lincosamide antibiotic drugs – **clindamycin**.[14]

- *Main indications:* staphylococcal infections particularly of bones and joints, endocarditis (heart valve infection); people who have an infection resistant to penicillin; bacterial infections of the vagina; mycoplasma pneumonia; lung abscess
- *Dosage and duration of treatment:* lincosamides are available as syrups, capsules, and in injection form. The medication should not be stopped before the end of the course or recurrence is likely, and also as this may encourage the evolution of resistant strains (survivors may 'learn' to defend against it another time).
- Bacterial resistance to the lincosamide antibiotics develops rapidly. It is found in around 25 percent of *Streptococcus aureus* as well as some streptococci in some parts of Europe, while in others (where the drug has not been much used) it is hardly present at all. Resistance is said to develop very rapidly once the drug is used, with resistant strains being found during the course of treatment when there were none at the start.

○ *Main common side-effects:* nausea, vomiting, diarrhea and, more rarely, rashes

○ *Main uncommon side-effects:* extremely serious *Pseudomembranous colitis*, which is caused by superinfection with *Clostridium difficile*. If colitis symptoms start, the medication is usually stopped immediately.

○ *Contraindications:* anyone with diarrhea or a history of colitis, liver or kidney disease will require special consideration as to whether the use of clindamycin is suitable; in general it probably will not be used in anyone with these histories or problems.

MACROLIDES

One of the main macrolide antibiotic now used is erythromycin. Others include clarithromycin and azithromycin.

○ The action of the macrolide antibiotics is similar to that of the tetracycline drugs (*see above*), since it achieves its effects by preventing the normal synthesis of protein by the bacteria which they are attacking, so preventing the bacteria from reproducing or surviving.

○ A major use of the macrolides is as alternatives to penicillin use when allergy exists towards this, and/or to treat:
  ○ infections of the chest in children, as well as
  ○ Legionnaires' disease
  ○ chronic prostate infections
  ○ intestinal infections involving Campylobacter
  ○ one of the macrolides, erythromycin, is used to prevent infections such as whooping cough.

○ Resistance to these drugs – especially by *Staphylococcus aureus* – was widespread, but newer versions of the macrolides have (for the moment) largely overcome this.

○ Mild and relatively common side-effects include nausea, vomiting, and diarrhea.
○ Dr Curtis Gemmel of Glasgow's Royal Infirmary and Glasgow Medical School, Scotland, reports that just like tetracycline (*see above*), erythromycin and others of this group of antibiotics weaken aspects of immune function.[15]
○ Most macrolide antibiotics cause few serious side-effects, aside from erythromycin, which can cause severe liver inflammation (hepatitis).

An example of the uses, cautions, and side-effects of one of the macrolide antibiotic drugs – **erythromycin**.[16]

○ *Main indications:* activity against a broad spectrum of bacteria involved in throat, middle ear, chest infections including rare pneumonias caused by mycoplasma. It is also used in Legionnaires' disease, gonorrhea, syphilis, diphtheria and in preventing the spread of whooping cough.
○ *Specific uses:* as an alternative to penicillin in people who are allergic to this. It is sometimes used to treat acne.
○ *Not normally prescribed for:* breastfeeding women. Infants require lower dosages.
○ *Dosage and duration of treatment:* by injection, capsule, tablet, or liquid; usually for no longer than 14 days (taken two to four times daily) as liver damage may result from taking this for any longer. The medication should not be stopped before the end of the course or recurrence is likely, and also as this may encourage the evolution of resistant strains (those that survive the medication because it is stopped too soon may 'learn' to defend against it another time).
○ *Main common side-effects:* nausea and vomiting, which is more likely when taken by mouth
○ *Main severe and relatively uncommon side-effects:* liver disease
○ *Long-term use* can lead to liver damage.

○ *Contraindications:* anyone with liver problems, previous allergy to erythromycin or who is taking other medications will require special consideration as to whether the use of erythromycin is suitable. Erythromycin and other macrolide antibiotics react with many other drugs, necessitating some important restrictions. They should not be used at the same time as theophylline (used in asthma and other bronchial conditions), carbamazepine (used in treatment of depression), warfarin (used to thin the blood in cardiovascular disease), digoxin (used to treat heart disease) or the antihistamine drugs terfenadine and astemizole (used in allergy).

IMIDAZOLES

Commonly used imidazoles include Flagyl (a metronidazole form of imidazole) and Fasigyn (a tinidazole form of imidazole).

○ The imidazole antibiotics are only active against bacteria which live without oxygen (anaerobic bacteria) and protozoa (one-celled microbes responsible for many tropical infections and diseases – usually resistant to most antibiotics).
○ The activity of these antibiotics is against a narrow range of target organisms (the opposite of broad-spectrum).
○ The use of imidazoles in bacterial infection is largely to treat conditions such as:
   ○ peritonitis
   ○ brain abscesses
   ○ pelvic abscess
   ○ deep wounds
   ○ protozoal infection such as amebic dysentery (caused by *Entamoeba histolyca*)
   ○ giardiasis (caused by *Giardia lamblia*)
   ○ vaginitis caused by *Trichomonas vaginalis*.

The action of the macrolide antibiotics is to interfere with the genetic material of the organism (DNA) and so prevent replication.

○ They are administered by mouth as tablets or liquids or by injection, drip infusion, or suppository.

○ Resistance to these drugs is rare.

○ Side-effects include nausea, vomiting, diarrhea, drowsiness, headaches. Upsets of the gastrointestinal tract can be reduced by taking the medication with food.

○ The urine may become discolored.

○ Long-term treatment or high dosages can lead to epileptic-like seizures and neuromuscular symptoms.

○ Metronidazole can cause severe liver problems and anyone with liver disease, or who is pregnant or breastfeeding should avoid these drugs.

An example of the uses, cautions, and side-effects of one of the imidazole antibiotic drugs – **metronidazole**.[17]

○ *Not normally prescribed for:* pregnant or breastfeeding women.

○ *Dosage and duration of treatment:* usually no longer than 10 days (5 days is more usual), by injection, tablet, liquid, or suppository (and as a gel) three times daily. The medication should not be stopped before the end of the course or recurrence is likely, and also as this may encourage the evolution of resistant strains (those that survive the medication because it is stopped too soon may 'learn' to defend against it another time).

○ *Special instructions:* avoid alcohol when this drug is being taken.

○ *Main common side-effects:* nausea, loss of appetite, diarrhea, and dark urine

○ *Main uncommon side-effects:* dry mouth with metallic taste, headache, dizziness and drowsiness, numbness and tingling (very rare)

○ *Long-term use* can lead to seizures and liver damage.

○ *Contraindications:* anyone with liver or kidney problems, a blood disorder, epilepsy or who is taking other medications will require special consideration as to whether the use of metronidazole is suitable. Anyone taking anticoagulant medication or lithium should be cautious regarding metronidazole; because of possible dizziness, caution is needed regarding driving and hazardous work. Alcohol must be avoided or flushing, nausea, vomiting, abdominal pain, and headache may result.

QUINOLONES

Commonly used quinolones include acrosoxacin, cinoxacin, ciprofloxacin and enoxacin.

○ The quinolone antibiotics were originally a narrow spectrum group of synthetic drugs which were found to have provoked resistance in many of their target organisms until the addition of fluorine into their structure.
○ In this way a newer generation of these drugs evolved called fluoroquinolones, which has, for the moment, reduced the degree of resistance and enormously broadened the spectrum of activity, so that they can be used in almost all areas of the body against a wide range of infective organisms.
○ Even newer developments include the marrying of the quinolone antibiotics with cephalosporins (*see above*), which has (again, for the moment, because as in all cases of antibiotic use, this will change in time) overcome resistance in some aggressive disease-causing organisms such as *Streptococcus pneumoniae*.
○ The effectiveness of the quinolone antibiotics is partly explained by their ability to inhibit enzymes associated with the genetic material of the bacteria (the DNA), so preventing the microorganism from reproducing itself. It achieves this without interfering with human DNA.

○ In addition, different antibiotics in this group of drugs have other means of damaging or killing bacteria, usually involving, in one way or another, the way the bacteria synthesize protein.

○ Having more than one means of killing or deactivating bacteria means that these drugs will probably maintain their effectiveness for longer than drugs which have only one method of attacking bacteria.

○ Quinolones are used in treatment of:
  ○ urinary, respiratory and gastrointestinal tract infections, as well as
  ○ gonorrhea
  ○ dysentery
  ○ skin infections.
  ○ The quinolone drugs are often used in patients allergic to penicillin-type antibiotics, or in cases where there is resistance to other antibiotics.

○ As mentioned, resistance to these drugs was widespread because of excessive early use; newer versions have (for the moment) largely reduced this. It has been found that when resistance develops against one of the quinolone drugs, the bacteria also become resistant to other antibiotics in this group.

○ Mild and relatively common side-effects affect around 10 percent of patients receiving quinolone drugs, and involve nausea, vomiting, and diarrhea, which sometimes becomes more serious with the development of *Pseudomembranous colitis*.

○ Most quinolone antibiotics cause few serious side-effects – about 1 person in 100 does, however, develop severe symptoms which might include anxiety, severe skin rash and itching, nightmares, and hallucinations, which usually stop when the drug is withdrawn.

○ Some versions known as trifluorinated quinolone antibiotics, such as fleroxacin, can cause relatively common photosensitivity (skin reaction to light), which can occur even weeks after use of the drug has been stopped.

○ Kidney failure has also been reported in some elderly patients receiving certain quinolone drugs (norfloxacin, ciprofloxacin).

○ Specific quinolones (pefloxacin, ciprofloxacin) have produced side-effects in young people (adolescents usually) involving severe arthritis-like joint problems.

An example of the uses, cautions, and side-effects of one of the quinolone antibiotic drugs – **ciprofloxacin**.[18]

○ *Main indications:* a wide range of applications but particularly useful in treatment of respiratory, urinary tract, and gastrointestinal infections. It is widely useful in the treatment of infections susceptible to penicillin in patients who have become allergic to penicillin.

○ *Not normally prescribed for:* pregnant women, breastfeeding women, infants and children.

○ *Dosage and duration of treatment:* a single dose is commonly prescribed for treatment of gonorrhea. Courses may be prolonged, as no significant dangers have emerged with long-term use, although the liver and kidneys may need to be monitored to ensure that no damage is taking place. Treatment is by injection (for severe systemic conditions) or more usually by tablets, taken twice daily. The medication should not be stopped before the end of the course or recurrence is likely, and also as this may encourage the evolution of resistant strains (those that survive the medication because it is stopped too soon may 'learn' to defend against it another time).

○ *Special instructions:* driving and hazardous work should be avoided during its use because of possible dizziness. Alcohol should be avoided during its use because of adverse side-effects. Drink plenty of fluids.

○ *Main common side-effects:* nausea, vomiting, diarrhea, and abdominal pain.
○ *Main uncommon side-effects:* dizziness, joint pain, headache, and skin rash.
○ *Long-term use* can lead to kidney or liver problems.
○ *Contraindications:* anyone with liver or kidney problems, or with a history of epilepsy, or who is taking other medications will require special consideration as to whether the use of ciprofloxacin is suitable.

Antibiotic Toxicity – Summary[19]

Dr. A. Ball, Senior Lecturer at St. Andrew's University in Scotland, reports the following forms and incidence of antibiotic-related side-effects:

Digestive Tract

○ Cephalosporins, penicillins, fluoroquinolones, macrolides, and some others cause mild to moderate nausea and abdominal discomfort.
○ In particular, erythromycin causes pain, nausea and vomiting in 16 percent of patients, with about half this number among patients receiving macrolide antibiotics.
○ Virtually all antibiotics are capable of producing *Pseudomembranous colitis.*
○ Between 10 and 25 percent of patients receiving clindamycin will develop diarrhea.
○ Between 5 and 10 percent of those receiving ampicillin develop diarrhea.
○ The development of diarrhea seems to result from either yeast (Candida) or bacterial (commonly *Clostridium difficile*) overgrowth when the normal flora is damaged. Toxins produced by

opportunistic bacterial activity including that of *Staphylococcus aureus* may also be to blame. This highlights the needs for strategies such as those listed in Chapters 9 and 10, to be followed by anyone taking antibiotics.

Liver Disease

○ Direct poisoning of the liver may occur with drugs such as isoniazid (for TB).
○ Allergic responses involving the liver are relatively common involving penicillin and cephalosporin antibiotics.
○ General liver disease can result from antibiotics such as the macrolides.
○ Tetracyclines can cause fatty changes in the liver, which is more likely when it is given intravenously, or in high doses, or to pregnant women.
○ Antibiotics such as erythromycin cause changes in liver function in 15 percent of cases treated, but 'only' 2 percent develop jaundice.
○ Fusidic acid (one of a class of antibiotics called Fusidanes, not reviewed in the lists above) commonly causes liver problems. Fortunately the jaundice is usually reversible.
○ Cotrimoxazole (*see Sulfa Drugs, above*) is a common cause of liver changes which are not severe enough to produce symptoms, and in some cases causes actual hepatitis.

Blood Diseases (such as Aplastic Anemia and Neutropenia)

○ Chloramphenicol, which is a widely used antibiotic for treatment of meningitis, brain abscesses and typhoid fever), can cause serious and even fatal blood disorders.

- Penicillin-like drugs used to treat staphylococcal infections can (rarely) cause neutropenia, which is a dramatic reduction in the number of white blood cells (neutrophils), which form the bulk of the first line of defense against infection.
- Penicillins, cephalosporins, sulphonamides and quinolones (and some other antibiotics) can cause severe blood diseases such as *Hemolytic anemia*.
- The antibiotic temafloxacin has been withdrawn from use because it has caused severe liver and kidney damage. Some of those affected also developed convulsions; a few died.
- The betalactam antibiotics (penicillins and cephalosporins) can sometimes (about 1 in 100 with the cephalosporins) cause problems in the way the blood clots, at times leading to excessive bleeding.
- Between 1 and 2 out of 100 patients receiving penicillins and cephalosporins (betalactams) develop thrombophlebitis (a blockage or 'clot', together with inflammation of a vein) – often at the site of the injection if this was the way the antibiotic was administered.
- Approximately 10 percent of people receiving erythromycin (*see discussion of the macrolide drugs, above*) also develop thrombophlebitis.

Central Nervous System Problems

- Excessive use of nalidixic acid (one of the quinolones) and metronidazole (one of the imidazole antibiotics, *see discussion above*) can cause convulsions.
- Excessive use of benzylpenicillin in certain circumstances, and/or administration of cephalosporin antibiotics intravenously or into the spinal cord, have led to convulsions and coma in rare cases.
- Damage to hearing has been associated with repeated or long courses of aminoglycosides antibiotics, and there are reports of hearing problems after only a single dose as well.

○ Cases of hearing damage and/or tinnitus (constantly hearing high-pitched noise) have been reported following high-dosage erythromycin and vancomycin use.

○ There are rare reports of confusion, hallucination, and delirium following use of fluoroquinolone antibiotics.

Allergy/Hypersensitivity

○ Most antibiotics, particularly penicillins and cephalosporins, can produce severe allergic reactions – involving rashes, swelling of the face and throat and other symptoms.

○ If this happens immediate medical attention is called for.

○ Once such a reaction occurs it is likely that all other drugs of that class are capable of producing a similar reaction.

○ Allergic reactions occur in very few patients, however just how serious, and how rare, this can be is indicated by the statistic that 2 people out of every 100,000 given penicillin are likely to die from such an allergic reaction.

○ Allergic skin rashes occur in 7 out of every 100 people receiving ampicillin and between 1 and 2 out of every 100 receiving intravenous cephalosporin medication.

○ Extreme sensitivity to light is possible with any of the quinolone drugs and with the tetracyclines.

Muscle and Joint Problems

○ Tetracyclines are contraindicated for children under 7 because of the effect they have on the teeth (staining them). If given to infants these drugs can cause short-term problems in bone formation.

○ Some of the quinolone drugs, including nalidixic acid and ciprofloxacin, can cause severe muscle damage and pain. Some of the penicillins have caused severe muscle inflammation.

Kidney and Liver Problems

○ Most antibiotics taken by mouth or injection have to be processed by the liver and excreted through the kidneys. They therefore need to be used very cautiously by anyone with existing or a history of problems of either the liver or the kidneys.
○ Erythromycin is particularly associated with liver problems.
○ The aminoglycosides are particularly likely to have negative effects on the kidneys.
○ The antibiotic vancomycin, kept in reserve for use on superbug infections, is particularly toxic for the kidneys, with approximately 5 out of every 100 patients receiving it developing serious problems. This is especially true if aminoglycoside antibiotics are being used at the same time.
○ Cotrimoxazole has a bad record for causing further kidney problems in people with any existing kidney disease.

Can Antibiotics Cause Cancer?

○ When tested in the laboratory, some of the antibiotics – notably metronidazole and the quinolones – can cause cells to mutate into potentially cancer-forming states in experimental animals. Careful monitoring in humans has failed to show any connection with cancer development when these drugs are used.

As indicated in the discussion of individual antibiotic types, particular attention needs to be given to the following groups when antibiotics are being prescribed:

○ pregnant or breastfeeding women
○ infants and young children
○ the elderly
○ people already receiving other medication (because of possible drug interactions)

Natural Alternatives to Antibiotics

○ anyone with a past allergic reaction to antibiotics
○ anyone with (or with a history of) kidney disease
○ anyone with (or with a history of) liver disease.

Conclusions and Suggestions

○ Antibiotics save lives.
○ Antibiotics can cause severe and sometimes unpredictable side-effects even when used correctly (right situation, right amount, etc.).
○ The effect on the internal ecology of the person receiving antibiotics is potentially devastating, long term, and is under-appreciated by doctors.
○ Antibiotics are over-used, misused, abused, and have become a major cause of ill-health.
○ Antibiotics are often used 'wrongly' in medicine – for example:
  ○ for patients who are not suitable to receive them (*see above*)
  ○ 'just in case' of a bacterial infection
  ○ against viral infections (when they are worse than useless)
  ○ against the wrong bacteria (i.e. ones they cannot effectively combat)
  ○ as broad-spectrum agents when the particular bacteria involved has not been identified – so encouraging resistance
  ○ in excessive amounts
  ○ in insufficient amounts
  ○ for too long a period
  ○ for too short a period
  ○ individually instead of in combination in specific circumstances.

The result is:

O widespread damage to the normal flora of the body and all that this can lead to in terms of illness
O increasing bacterial resistance leading to virtually untreatable infections.

The conclusion we need to draw from this is that unless there is a change in attitude toward infectious disease, with greater emphasis on hygiene and natural immunity, whether through the methods outlined in later chapters or by other means such as immunization (which carries its own risks and dangers), we are heading for a crisis which could overwhelm the medical profession as it attempts to deal with superbug infections in hospitals and the community.

5: Immune Enhancement: Lifestyle, Detoxification, and Mind-Body Factors

Some of the many ways in which the natural defenses of your immune system can be weakened are discussed in this chapter.

This does not have to happen. You can do something – in fact a lot – about preventing your immune system from being overloaded, weakened, or damaged. Even if it already is weakened, there is still a great deal you can do about repairing and improving its abilities to defend you against both external attack – from bacteria, viruses, etc. – and from internal damage which can lead to serious ill-health.

Where Is the Immune System?

The immune system is not just one system like the digestive or nervous or circulatory systems, in fact it includes all three of these as part of its 'machinery,' along with most organs of the body, the brain, the skin, the hormonal system, and much more. To a large extent you are your immune system, or rather aspects of it are found almost everywhere in the body.

The part of the immune system in which we are interested provides immediate protection from infection, and before we look at ways of making this vital self-regulating facet of the body more efficient we need to have a basic understanding of it.

WHAT HAPPENS WHEN WE ARE ILL?

○ If you cut yourself you heal.
○ If you break a bone it will usually mend.
○ When you are reasonably healthy, infections are almost always self-limiting, which means that your defense system takes care of the invader.

These are all examples of a process called homeostasis – the self-regulating, self-healing, self-repairing mechanism that works day and night to defend and to restore or maintain health without outside instruction, integrated and coordinated by means of the brain, the hormonal system, and the nervous system, as well as by means of hundreds of chemical messengers which are used to give instructions that control the reactions of the body to invasion and damage.

Infection, injury, allergy, stress – all of these are corrected or coped with automatically by our defense system when it is in good working order.

But when anyone's immune system is not functioning efficiently, when it has been compromised or damaged or where the number of things it is being asked to handle are just too numerous and perhaps overwhelming (possibly involving emotional stress, infections, toxicity, deficiency, allergy as well as other stressors – whether chemical, physical or emotional – all at once), help is needed – treatment of one sort or another is called for.[1]

If it is to be successful in restoring health, any treatment needs to either:

○ support and help the natural defenses of the body – or
○ remove some of the stresses and strains with which it is coping – or
○ do both of these – most importantly, while avoiding causing additional problems which might actually make matters worse.[2]

A treatment which efficiently helps in one way, but which makes matters worse in another, is obviously of doubtful value.

Good and Bad Treatment

If you develop a headache because your reading glasses are not the correct prescription for your eyes, taking a painkilling tablet to ease the headache may help the pain but does not resolve the underlying problem.

The headache will recur, and if the tablet also produces abdominal bleeding (aspirin, for example) then you have not dealt with the cause, *and* you have created a new health problem as well.

If you have your eyes checked and get the correct reading glasses, the headaches will cease and no new problems will have been created.

But what if the headache was really bad and you needed relief before you could get your eyes tested?

A safer way of easing the head pain might have been available (eye exercises, massage, relaxation methods, herbal medicine, etc.), any one of which could ease your symptoms while not loading you with yet another health problem.

Ask yourself which is good medicine and which is bad in this example?

If you start to vomit and develop diarrhea after eating something which is 'off,' should you do anything to stop the diarrhea and the vomiting?

If you do, you will be halting the very processes which are trying to get the toxic material out of your body. Does this mean that you should do nothing at all?

No, because in such a situation, especially in children, maintaining fluid levels is vital and there are times when the reaction to the toxin or poison is actually causing harm. This is where good medical advice is called for. However, in most instances, keeping as comfortable as possible, maintaining fluid levels and doing nothing to stop the elimination is the best approach.

In this example the symptoms which our instincts tell us should be controlled are in fact the best 'treatment' we can have. The body is doing what it was designed to do: protecting itself.

If an actual dangerous microorganism were involved in this 'food poisoning,' then an antibiotic might indeed be called for. However, alternatives do exist, as will be explained. Even if antibiotics are needed, strategies exist for ensuring that any damage they may cause will be minimal (*see Chapter 9*).

ANTIBIOTICS ARE NOT ALWAYS GOOD MEDICINE

Unfortunately the main drug treatments used to deal with infection – antibiotics – often fit exactly into the frame of 'bad medicine,' because although they may do a good job of retarding aspects of bacterial activity (*see Chapters 1, 2, 3 and 4*), this is at such a cost (in terms of the new health problems caused) that it pays us to seek safer alternatives unless the use of antibiotics is truly vital.

Healing Comes from Within

Even when a method of treatment is safe, harmless, and helpful, it is never the treatment itself which makes you better, but simply the fact that an opportunity has been created for the body to normalize itself once again – for homeostasis to operate, for the immune system to do what it was designed to do.

So as we look at the list of what can depress the immune system (*see page 97*), and start to survey the options we have to help ourselves boost immune function, we need to keep in mind the fact that our goal is to improve the efficiency of these self-healing mechanisms and systems so that they can operate more efficiently while also removing as much of the burden the body is coping with physically or emotionally.

SYMPTOMS ARE NOT ALL BAD

It is also important to recognize that sometimes symptoms are just evidence of healing in progress, as in the food poisoning example above.

When you have a temperature, this is a signal that your immune system is dealing with a necessary task, possibly fighting against an invading microorganism.

Most bacteria and viruses die when heated, and this is happening when your temperature rises to 38°C (100°F) or higher.

As we will see later in this chapter when we look at hydrotherapy methods, hyperthermia (artificial fever therapy) is an approach that actually tries to raise core body temperature in order to help kill bacteria and viruses.[3]

Unfortunately, in the everyday world the first thing many people do when they have a fever is to try to bring it down – by use of aspirin or other similar drugs, or by demanding an antibiotic from their doctor.

There is an almost immediate attitude to symptoms such as a fever: 'It hurts, or is unpleasant, therefore I must get rid of it.'

But the fever *is* the treatment. It is the evidence that the body is dealing with the infection. And, in almost all cases, unless health is really compromised or the fever gets out of control (very rare), it gets better on its own.

Another irony is that fevers which are a response to an infection usually get better faster when they are not treated by drugs which push the temperature down. All this does, in most cases, is to drag the process out for longer.

So it is important that we try to overcome the sort of response in which symptoms are treated without thought, so that they are only interfered with if they are dangerous or severe.

And of course anything which treats symptoms (say pain or infection) must try not to make other aspects of the person's recovery more difficult (say by increasing the toxic load or interfering with any of the body's systems).

Remember that in good health you are usually resistant to most infections and your body will deal with them on its own – without help – if some basic 'rules' are followed which support immune function.

The summary below shows those aspects of our immune function which are involved in offering 'resistance'; following this a list of some of the many ways in which these defenses can be weakened.

Simplified Sequence of Infection

○ An invading bacteria enters the body – we call this invader an antigen.
○ A defense cell called a macrophage 'eats' the invading bacteria but retains some of the proteins on its surface.
○ The macrophage carries these protein 'markers' to lymphoid tissue (the tonsils or spleen, for example), where T-lymphocyte cells read these and recognize that they are 'foreign.'
○ This causes an alarm – a recognition that a defensive response against an enemy is called for. So the T-cell multiplies and produces different versions of itself. These are:
  1 memory cells – which remember past infections or the characteristics of the present invader – and so are able to recognize and attack it
  2 natural killer cells – which are used to attack bacterial invaders directly
  3 suppressor cells – which help to control and calm these defense reactions so that they do not get out of hand
  4 helper cells (B-lymphocytes) – which stimulate lymph tissues (such as the tonsils and the spleen) to produce what are called 'antigen specific B-lymphocytes' which manufacture immunoglobulins (Ig) to neutralize toxins secreted by bacterial invaders as well as helping make them more vulnerable to attack.

○ In this way the body builds up specific defenses against invaders so that the T-cells can repulse and overwhelm them.
○ After the infection is over, the body is left with a built-in memory of the invader so that it will be recognized if it tries to invade again, and so be dealt with efficiently, usually without symptoms such as a fever, which might have been part of the body's first-time reaction to the infection.

The Components of Immune Function

These are the main immune organs that defend you:

○ The lymph nodes, such as the tonsils, where
  ○ lymphocytes are made, and stored
  ○ foreign proteins are 'consumed' by the macrophages

○ The spleen, where
  ○ lymphocytes are produced
  ○ macrophages consume both foreign invaders and used-up blood cells
  ○ red blood cells are stored for future use

○ The thymus gland, where
  ○ T-lymphocytes are produced
  ○ thymus hormones are produced.

The cells which are part of immune function include:

○ Neutrophils – which make up between 50 and 75 percent of the total number of white blood cells, and which attack and consume bacterial invaders as well as waste material in the bloodstream. They also release chemicals which can help control bacteria. These neutrophils are manufactured in the bone marrow.

○ Lymphocytes – which comprise around 25 to 40 percent of the white blood cells, and are either T-cells (from the thymus) or B-cells (from the bone marrow). The lymphocytes carry out many of the same roles as the neutrophils.

○ Eosinophils – which make up between 1 and 4 percent of white blood cells – are made in the bone marrow and have a role in controlling inflammatory processes. Their numbers increase in some allergic conditions.

○ Basophils – which make up just 1 percent of white blood cells and which release histamine (among other things), involved in allergic and inflammatory reactions.

○ Monocytes make up the balance of white blood cells (3 to 6 percent). They are made in the bone marrow and are the early stages of the macrophages.

○ Plasma cells are made in the lymphoid tissues (spleen, tonsils, etc.) as well as by B-cells which manufacture antibodies (*see above*).

○ Macrophages, which are formed from monocytes, 'eat' cell debris and foreign material. In general they help in the immune response to invasion.

○ Mast cells are very similar to basophils, from which they are made, but they are found not just in the bloodstream but throughout the body. They release histamine as part of allergic and inflammatory responses.

These, then, are the main players in immune defense. They can, for numerous reasons, become weakened – as we will see later in this chapter.

It is when invading organisms take advantage of a 'weakened' immune system that they cause what are called 'opportunistic' infections. When opportunistic infections occur it is almost always because immune function has been partially overwhelmed in the face of having to cope with nutritional, toxic, emotional, and infectious stresses.

T-4 and B-lymphocytes and other aspects of our first-line defenses may, by the time a bacteria invades, be in short supply. Other aspects of the body's defenses may also be compromised, perhaps as a result of enzyme deficiencies in the liver, kidney, digestive tract and/or lungs, or because of hormonal imbalances and dysfunction.

Many of these situations can be helped and reversed using a host of possible interventions, as will be discussed in this and the next chapter.

A double thrust to any intervention could involve both immune support (helping it get well again) and a direct method of killing infection of whatever sort, literally taking over the role of the immune system for a while in this particular regard.

This is of course what antibiotics try to do, and at times this is the best choice. However, if safer alternatives are available and antibiotics are not judged to be absolutely essential, then knowing what these alternatives are is vital.

FACTORS THAT WEAKEN THE BODY'S DEFENSES

First let's look at what has been shown by research to be able to weaken the immune system:[4]

> **Sugar:** Consuming 90 g of honey or fruit sugar (or fruit juice) or regular sucrose will cause a drop by up to 50 percent in white blood cell activity for between one and five hours.
>
> **Alcohol:** Sufficient alcohol to cause intoxication depresses white blood cell action as well as slowing down neutrophil activity. Alcohol consumption causes vitamin and mineral deficiency, specifically of folic acid, thiamine, vitamin B_6, vitamin A, vitamin C, zinc, magnesium, and potassium. T- and B-lymphocytes including natural killer cells decline in number when alcohol is consumed in anything but extremely small quantities (even the equivalent of $1\frac{1}{2}$ glasses of wine daily makes infection more likely).

The alcohol in one glass of wine, one beer, or one shot of liquor can cut your white cells' antibody production in half for 24 hours. Alcohol also provokes what is known as free-radical oxidation, an important phenomenon which is explained later in this chapter.[5]

Allergic reaction: When the body is reacting to a food or substance in an allergic way, immune function is diverted away from antibacterial surveillance and activity. The allergic reaction also results in increased toxic debris which can damage immune function further.

Toxicity: as occurs after exposure to pesticides, heavy metals (lead, mercury, cadmium, etc.) as well as petrochemicals, ozone, sulfur dioxide, organic solvents, and silicone implants – leads to

- O reduction in the formation of antibodies
- O less efficient bacteria-killing white blood cell activity
- O damage to protective mucous membranes (and so increased chance of infection) – some of these ill-effects are the result of direct toxicity (poisoning) and some are caused by oxidation processes, a brief explanation of which is given later in this chapter
- O decreased natural killer cell activity
- O depressed T and B cell production and activity
- O damage to the thymus gland.

Medical drugs (especially steroids such as cortisone): Many commonly used drugs, including aspirin, reduce antibody production and suppress immune function. Steroid medications (cortisone, hydrocortisone, prednisone, etc.) are commonly used in the treatment of various common illnesses (arthritis, for example). These are extremely quick-acting drugs and can give marked symptom relief. Balancing this is the fact that without exception they are immune depressants, producing a rapid decline in T and B cell numbers, reducing cell-mediated immunity and making infection much easier to acquire, as well as having other negative influences on the body.

Smoking: Tobacco is a known depressant of immune function. Anyone who wishes to protect or improve immune function should avoid smoking completely, as well as the company of people who smoke. The smoke and tar from one cigarette can severely compromise your white cell activity for 24 hours. Cigarette smoke also contains enormous quantities of free radicals which cause oxidation.

Stimulant drugs including amphetamines, cocaine, and various forms to psychedelic drugs such as LSD. All depress immune function. Cocaine is the most addictive of these and its use produces extreme anxiety states which often lead to the use of other drugs such as alcohol, opioids, and marijuana – with severe immune-depressing results.[6]

Antibiotics: When used excessively there is a general immune weakening, a likelihood of yeast overgrowth in the intestines and (as discussed in Chapter 8) the chance of increasing resistance by microorganisms so that they become harder to overcome.

Candida (yeast) infection of the bowel: The toxins formed by yeast when this inhabits sections of the bowel and friendly bacteria have been weakened (perhaps due to antibiotics) suppress immune function.

Vaccination: When a vaccination is given the body's defenses are mobilized to deal with this assault, and as a result overall protective activity is depressed for the next several weeks.

Emotional stress: When emotionally stressed, *all* aspects of immune function are depressed. In particular the thymus gland is affected, with resulting depression of T-cell production and activity. It has been proven by the science of psychoneuroimmunology, which examines the links between the mind, the nervous system and the immune system, that emotional stress can suppress aspects of immune function by up to 60 percent. Controlling or eliminating stress is one of the greatest anchors of health.

Hormonal imbalance (e.g. at menopause): While the body is adapting to the major changes in hormone production that follow the onset of menopause, immune function is less efficient.

Too much exercise: Excessive exercise leads to increased demands on repair functions and a loss of overall immune activity.

Too little rest: Natural killer cell activity is reduced when inadequate rest is taken.

Nutritional deficiencies (notably of the main B-complex vitamins, vitamins A, C, E, and the minerals selenium and zinc): When a nutritional deficiency exists – something which is widespread in all sections of society – *all* aspects of immune function are depressed.

Severe injury: Because of the inflammation and repair activity involved in severe trauma, other aspects of the immune defense capacity are weakened.

Chronic infection: When infections are common and/or lengthy, immune function can be overwhelmed.

Obesity: Antibody production and white blood cell activity are reduced in people who are severely overweight.

How to Know If Your Immune System Is Not as Efficient as It Should Be

The following general signs should alert you:

Excessive tiredness	If the degree of your fatigue is not directly related to the amount of activity in your life, your immune system may be under-functioning.
Frequent infections	Colds, sore throats, sinus problems, etc.

	Are you someone who catches every cold that seems to be going around?
Infections and inflammations which linger	Whether the result of a virus (e.g. herpes), yeast infection (e.g. candidiasis/ thrush, athlete's foot, fungal nails, etc.), parasite activity or something else altogether. Do you have infections, however mild, which never seem to go away?
Cuts and grazes which are slow to heal	Are these still unhealed weeks after they happen?
A history of malignant disease	Is there a strong family history (or a previous history of your own) of cancer?
Chronic allergies	Are you someone who is regularly reacting to something, whether a food, a chemical or a pollen? Or do you 'always' have a slight runny nose (allergic rhinitis)?

WHAT SHOULD YOU DO IF IMMUNE FUNCTION IS DEPRESSED?

○ Be alert to how your bodily defenses and repair systems are working.

○ Look at the possible factors which can weaken immune function as listed above – and see how many (if any) apply to you.

○ If any of them do apply to you – do something about it. Read the advice here and in Chapters 6 and 9. There can be no more important aspect of health protection than making your natural defenses more efficient.

METHODS

Fortunately, a wide range of methods have been shown to be useful in achieving these objectives.[7]

These options include:

○ Nutritional intervention – probably the single most impor-tant aspect of any concerted effort to restore immune function (*see Chapter 6*). This might involve detoxification efforts, replenishing deficient nutrients, or attempts to help control oxidation processes (*see below*) which place increased demands on the body's defense and repair mechanisms.

○ Use of 'friendly bacteria' – probiotics – to help the almost always damaged bowel function of anyone who is immune-compromised (*see also Chapter 9*).

○ Use of safe non-toxic herbal medications as an alternative to drugs, since the latter can cause further stress to the immune system (*see Chapter 6*).

○ Hydrotherapy hyperthermia (raising core body temper-ature by use of hydrotherapy methods), which you may wish to try if it seems to offer a useful aid – *see Chapter 6*.

○ Lifestyle modification (exercise, quitting smoking, etc.) as well as detoxification approaches including fasting (to be discussed later in this chapter) – all useful strategies for improving immune function.

○ Mind-centered approaches such as deep relaxation and visualization methods (this chapter), which can make a sound immune system work even better and can help restore a weakened one.

○ Acupuncture for symptomatic control and for balancing internal energy patterns (*Chapter 6*).

Oxidation and Free Radical Activity

When your white blood cells defend against invading micro-organisms, they produce minute amounts of hydrogen peroxide – the same material used to bleach hair. This is highly toxic and damaging to the bacteria and will often kill it. So that the cells of the body itself are not damaged by this material, it is usually rapidly 'quenched' by antioxidants such as vitamins A, E and C, and the minerals selenium or zinc in the bloodstream or tissues.

When you injure yourself and inflammation results, part of the process involves the release from tissues, where they are stored, of metals such as copper or iron. These then produce different types of 'free radicals' – molecules with a free attachment arm – which are used in the inflammation process as part of the healing effort.

We can see in these two examples that your body has learned to use the process of free radical oxidation to help itself. This is a process which we can see in everyday life, as you can illustrate for yourself by carrying out the following experiment:

- Cut an apple or potato in half. Squeeze the juice of a lemon onto one exposed half; leave the other half alone.
- Watch what happens over a period of minutes: the half with the lemon juice stays white; the other half turns brown.
- What you have seen is the action of oxygen in the air, which contains free radical molecules (explained further below) on the browned apple/potato. You have also seen how antioxidants such as vitamin C (in the lemon juice) can 'quench' this process.

When rubber perishes, metal rusts or your skin ages and wrinkles, or when fat becomes rancid – you are observing the same process: oxidation.

When hair is bleached with hydrogen peroxide (H_2O_2) you are seeing the same process but in a speeded-up format, because H_2O_2 is a highly active oxidation material.

WHAT IS A FREE RADICAL?

Not, to be sure, a terrorist who is out of jail. Let us go back to H_2O_2.

O Each atom of Hydrogen (H) has 1 attachment arm.

O Each atom of Oxygen (O) has 2 attachment arms.

O If we put 2 hydrogen atoms (H_2) together with 1 oxygen atom (O) – that is, 1 hydrogen for each free oxygen arm – we have H_2O: water. All the 'arms' of the oxygen atom are occupied by a hydrogen atom in this stable combination, which is called a molecule. There are no free arms.

O If, however, we put 2 hydrogen atoms (H_2) together with 2 oxygen atoms (O_2), we are left with 2 free arms in the resulting hydrogen peroxide molecule – H_2O_2. These free arms are what makes the H_2O_2 molecule capable of causing so much damage. It is why bleach (H_2O_2) can grab hold of cells in normal tissues such as hair and change them, altering their color and texture.

O This also explains the severe tissue damage that may occur when the fats in the body, in each cell, are attacked by free radicals (produced by excessive heavy metal toxicity, pesticides or cigarette smoke, for example). And this is far more likely when we are deficient in the normal antioxidants which we are supposed to obtain from our food.

So a combination of too many free radicals (pollution, toxicity, high fat levels, etc. in the body) and too few antioxidant nutrients (vitamins A, C, E, selenium, zinc, certain amino acids, etc.) can cause damage which makes enormous demands on the defense and repair mechanisms of the body.

What Causes Free Radicals to Be Released in the Body?

○ injury (trauma)
○ burns
○ extreme cold
○ excessive exercise
○ blood supply deficiency to tissues (ischemia)
○ inflammation
○ infection
○ exposure to radiation.

If there also is a deficiency of antioxidants, these processes may become prolonged. So when inflammation continues for a longer time than is normal, or injured tissues are very slow to heal, free radical oxidation may be partly to blame.

The following conditions/diseases are associated with (not all necessarily caused by it, but certainly encouraged by) free radical activity:

○ arthritis
○ arteriosclerosis
○ cancer
○ cardiovascular conditions such as myocardial infarct
○ cataracts
○ cirrhosis of the liver
○ degenerative diseases of the brain and nervous system such as Parkinson's disease and Alzheimer's disease
○ emphysema
○ inflammatory bowel disease
○ kidney diseases such as nephrotoxicity
○ stroke
○ viral diseases

and many more...

WHAT CAN YOU DO ABOUT FREE RADICAL OXIDATION?

Many of the methods for enhancing immune function and detoxification (described in the rest of this chapter and the next) will significantly reduce a tendency toward free radical activity, and therefore the demands on immune function.

The Aims of the Advice

Some of the methods explained below can be directed toward overall immune enhancement; others are more useful in trying to halt infection; some are capable of doing both. Read the notes which follow – see which aspects apply to you and which methods appeal to you, so that you can make choices based on information rather than guesswork.

Lifestyle (Exercise and Habits) and Immune Function

'Lifestyle' means just about everything we do, think and feel daily as we go about our lives, which impacts on our health. So one major area of self-help for the immune system lies in alterations we can make to our personal lifestyle.

Changing to a lifestyle that is health-supportive has definite immune-enhancing effects – for example, giving up smoking and reducing excessive alcohol consumption and/or the use of drugs will help the immune system to become stronger.

Improving nutrition and supplementing the diet has been shown to be of great help to people with compromised immune systems – see detailed advice below.[8]

Changing from negative to positive mental attitudes has proven immune-enhancing effects – due to the direct link between the immune system and the mind, as proved by studies in what is known as psychoneuroimmunology (*see below*).

Aspects of our spirituality also fall into this all-embracing area of what we do, believe, and feel – all of which can be shown to influence our immune systems and general health – for better or worse.[9]

Lifestyle factors prepare the soil into which infections are planted; how well these thrive and how sick they make us depend largely on the environment in which they find themselves. This can be influenced by how toxic we may be as well as whether or not we are nutritionally deficient, and also by the influence of a wide range of mental/emotional factors impacting on the immune system.[10] This 'soil,' our body/mind complex in which any infection is acting, will naturally enough also be dramatically influenced by the way previous illnesses have been treated, the drugs and surgical procedures used, and the residues of unresolved health problems which we may carry.[11]

Hans Selye, the great Canadian researcher, has shown that single stress factors are reasonably easy for an intact defense system to handle. But when there are two, three … ten – or more – stress factors, the cumulative effect is to overwhelm the potential for maintaining health, or recovering it. These 'stress factors' need to be addressed; if at least some can be ameliorated – by getting enough sleep and rest, by learning relaxation methods and stress-coping strategies, by improving the diet and encouraging detoxification – in short by doing whatever can be done using the best of orthodox and/or alternative methods to deal with infections and other health problems – the chances of relative or complete success are made greater.[12]

PSYCHONEUROIMMUNOLOGY

Experience in the field of cancer has shown just how important a part the mind can play in recovery.[13] Research to date into the area of psychoneuroimmunology (PNI) has come to three basic conclusions:[14]

1 The mind and body are intimately connected, and this connection also involves a direct link between the mind and the immune system (using the nervous and the hormonal systems as linking mechanisms).

2 The defense of the body (immune system) is directly linked to the thoughts and emotions of the individual.

3 Hormonal and nervous system control over the defenses of the body (including immune function) is profound.

MIND ISSUES AS PART OF COMBINED IMMUNE SUPPORT

In a one-year study at Bastyr University, Seattle, a combination of nutritional, herbal, homeopathic, hydrotherapeutic, psychological counseling and other methods were employed to treat people with severe immune depression. As part of this overall healing approach there was also a major emphasis on psychological support. Patients were requested to begin some form of individual or group psychotherapeutic process if not already doing so. A support group met weekly and focused on open discussion of emotional, physical and spiritual issues as well as meditation and positive affirmation strategies.[15]

Dr. Herb Joiner-Bey of Seattle says, 'Without spiritual and mental involvement people find it difficult to generate the commitment to getting themselves well.'[16]

Robert Cathcart, MD (developer of a method for Vitamin C treatment of immune depression – *see Chapter 6*) puts it succinctly: 'All the vitamin C in the world won't make up for a lousy attitude.'

These thoughts can be translated into very precise, scientifically measurable effects. For example, one study showed that when stressed by exams some students show specific decline in immune system defenses (decline in natural killer cell activity, for example) which allows for decreased resistance to infection.[17]

This is important news – but even more important is the conclusion which this medical research came to, based on the fact that not all students show such poor responses: 'The negative immune system changes (mitogen and natural killer cell activity decline) imply that *it is the individual's response to stress that determines the effect on immunity, rather than the stress itself.'*

What we 'think about' the things that happen to us matters far, far, more than the events themselves.

The key conclusion, therefore, is that if emotions and attitudes can negatively influence the immune system, then these mind-based influences can also do the opposite – help restore immune function.

HOW TO HELP YOURSELF

Anything which reduces negative influences on the nervous system, whether relaxation, meditation or visualization (guided imagery), bodywork (massage) or acupuncture, or some form of psychotherapeutic counseling/treatment/group work – anything which leads to a 'distress-free' state of mind – will help immune function.

This is quite a menu of methods from which to choose, a veritable catalogue of possibilities, one of which is bound to suit you. Whether counseling, stress-coping strategies, deep relaxation methods, meditation and visualization – or any other method – is used doesn't matter, just so long as it 'feels right' to the person involved and does no harm while underlying stresses are resolved.[18]

What is vital is that the mind and the emotions should not be neglected as the more obviously practical methods of nutrition and medication or other therapeutic intervention come into play.

Methods such as deep relaxation, meditation, guided imagery, and visualization are all taught as part of the recovery protocol at centers such as the UK's Bristol Cancer Help Centre, and these methods have now been adopted by many mainstream medical cancer clinics and hospitals – because they offer very real benefits in terms of survival.

Just as stress can produce a negative impact on defense mechanisms, relaxation or other stress-coping strategies can produce immune enhancement. This book is not the place to outline the actual methods, but if you wish to do the best you can for your immune system you should seek out organizations and teachers who can instruct and guide you toward the best of these methods for your own regular use.

Detoxification/Fasting and Immune Function

FASTING FOR HEALTH

When you stop eating (but keep up liquid intake) for 24 to 48 hours, some amazing changes take place in the body, including a dramatic improvement in immune function:[19]

○ Macrophage activity increases, boosting defenses.
○ Cell-mediated immunity is improved (T-lymphocyte activity, for example).
○ There is a decrease (a detoxification) in levels of undesirable antigen-antibody complexes which are the debris of previous immune activity.
○ Increases are seen in immunoglobulin levels (which neutralize toxins secreted by bacterial invaders, as well as helping to make the bacteria more vulnerable to attack).
○ Neutrophil antibacterial activity increases.
○ Monocytes' ability to kill bacteria improves.
○ Natural killer cell activity is much enhanced.
○ Detoxification by the white cells increases.
○ Antioxidant damage reduces and free radical levels drop.
○ …other benefits include improved status of mucous membranes, reducing the chance of infection.

Fasting is one of the oldest methods of healing. It is instinctive in sick animals and probably was in primitive humans, too.

If carried out sensibly, fasting can be useful in both treating and preventing disease.

Fasting is often confused with starvation, but strictly speaking it is abstinence for a given time from solid food, but not from liquids.

Some experts say fasting is effective only if water is the only liquid taken during the fast, whereas others advocate the use of vegetable juices. Opinion also differs on how long a fast should continue: this depends largely on whether it is being used to treat ill-health or as a method of preventive medicine, to improve well-being and enhance immune function.

No one should attempt a long fast (more than three days) unless they are under the supervision of an experienced practitioner.

Fasting is useful in most cases of physical illness, but there are certain circumstances where it should not be used without qualified supervision. Anyone –

○ with an ulcer
○ with a history of gout
○ who is pregnant
○ who has diabetes
○ who has heart disease which requires constant medication
○ who is regularly taking steroid medication (cortisone, for example)
○ who has kidney disease
○ who has cancer
○ who has an eating disorder of any sort
○ who is afraid of the idea of fasting

– should seek professional advice before trying any self-treatment with fasting.

In most of these conditions fasting can be helpful, but needs to be monitored and supervised in case of unusual reactions, especially if the person undertaking the fast is or has been on regular medication.

This warning does not mean that fasting is unsuitable for people with these conditions, but it does mean that expert help is required to decide on the type of fast and for how long it should be maintained.

Some odd things might happen to the body during a fast as toxic debris is released. It is best to understand what might happen before beginning a fast, so that you don't worry overmuch when it does happen. The 'symptoms of fasting' are not serious and are often no more than signs of detoxification in action. The sort of signs you can expect to notice are:

○ a furred tongue
○ bad breath
○ feeling colder than usual
○ feeling 'flu-like' symptoms
○ headache and nausea
○ production of dark and often offensive urine
○ (and sometimes) the voiding of amazing accretions from the bowels.

The degree and intensity of these signs of the body cleansing itself of accumulated toxic waste will vary greatly from person to person, often depending on the underlying health and vitality of the individual, as well as the type of fast being used.

Surprisingly, hunger is often not noticed after the first day.

Fasting can be seen as a preparation for spontaneous self-healing by the body. It is not a 'cure' for anything in particular but provides the body with a chance to eliminate toxins which may be preventing the body from functioning normally or healing itself, while at the same time increasing the efficiency of the immune system's defense activities.

This is why it is important not to treat the initial signs of fasting, such as a 'sick' headache, with any drugs or potions that will suppress them – as this will compromise the benefits being generated by the fast.

The headache will pass, and the tongue will become pink and healthy again, after the fast. All the other symptoms which are the result of the fast will disappear too.

A short fast may not be long enough for all these symptoms to appear, and with repetition their intensity will decrease until, in time, fasts may be enjoyed without marked symptoms and with a noticeable change in health in terms of energy and clarity of mind.

Colonic Irrigation?

An area of controversy in fasting is the use of enemas, colonic irrigation, and laxatives.

There are times when one of these may be called for. If, however, there is no history of constipation and the individual's general health is good, then washing out the bowel is seldom necessary during or after a fast.

If a chronic illness is involved, especially of the bowel, or if there is a chronic allergic or catarrhal condition, then there is a good case for periodic enemas or a herbal laxative being given before and after a short fast.

There are no rigid rules regarding this, but it is important to recognize that the state of health of the bowel largely decides the degree of health of the body.

Health is impossible without a healthy digestive system, and fasting is one of the best ways of improving this.

Supplements During the Fast?

Supplements of 'friendly' bacteria (*acidophilus* and *bifidus* – *see Chapter 9*) are a definite aid to healthy digestion and internal detoxification, especially during a period of intense detoxification activity such as a fast.

These bacterial cultures are therefore recommended during the fast. No other supplements should be taken during this period of 'physiological rest.'

During and After the Fast

Breaking the fast correctly is also important. After any length of time without solid food there must be a gentle transition back to a full diet (*see notes on page 117*).

It is also important that during a fast some exercise is taken; staying in bed is seldom called for, but plenty of rest and relaxation are useful. So it is unwise to fast while carrying on normal work.

It is also unwise, and contraindicated, to drive during a fast because dizziness may occur.

Fresh air and rest are important, as is the avoidance of stress, which helps to explain the popularity of health farms and hydros, which can offer a restful environment and pleasant diversions such as massage and hydrotherapy during this period of detoxification.

How Often and How Long Should You Fast?

Three-day fasts, undertaken over a weekend, are a good introduction to the experience, and the details of such an exercise have been set out and described below.

It is necessary to set aside a weekend for such fasting, during which you drop all major obligations and duties.

A three-day detoxification every four to six weeks, over six or twelve months, will provide a dramatic improvement in health in most people.

Alternatively, you might prefer to fast for one day each week.

Method:

- ○ A light meal can be eaten midday on a Saturday, followed by juice only from Saturday evening through to Sunday evening.
- ○ The fast can be broken Sunday evening or Monday morning.

○ This 24- to 36-hour fast every week or fortnight will be extremely beneficial to health.

In all cases the aim of a fast is to rest the body from the constant need to digest and process food.

The principles involved in fasting can also be applied to everyday eating to make us feel more vital and lively. For instance, breakfast implies that we have been, for a period, without food. This is literally true if the last meal of the previous day was at 6 p.m. and breakfast is at 7 or 8 a.m. next day. But if we eat after 9 at night then the digestive system will barely have finished coping with the evening meal before the next food starts to arrive. Such a pattern of eating makes people feel sluggish and lethargic.

By eating earlier in the evening, with no snacks later on, you can be livelier in the morning and have a rested digestive system ready for the next day.

Remember, longer fasts should only be undertaken with the help of a qualified nutritionally-oriented health care practitioner, although a short – 24- to 72-hour – fast is safe to apply without supervision unless contraindicated (*see list above*).

Preparing for a Fast

The day before: an herbal laxative such as psyllium seeds, a broth made of flax seed (linseed), or castor oil should be taken after the midday meal, which should itself be light (vegetarian for preference, such as a mixed salad or a vegetable soup).

In the evening: have a light fruit meal including pears, apple or grapes, or instead of fruit have a vegetable broth – see recipe below.

Vegetable Broth Recipe

○ Use organically grown vegetables if possible. If not, scrub vegetables well before use.

- Into 10 cups of spring water, place 4 cups of finely chopped beetroot, carrots, thick potato peelings, parsley, zucchini and leaves of beetroot or parsnips.
- Use no sulfur-rich vegetables such as cabbages or onions, which might produce gas.
- Simmer for 5 minutes over a low heat to allow for the breakdown of the vegetable fiber and the release of nutrients into the liquid.
- Cool and strain, using only the liquid and not the left-over vegetable content.
- Don't add salt, as this broth will contain ample natural minerals which are rapidly absorbed by the body, thus providing nutrients without straining the digestive system.
- This broth is alkaline and neutralizes any acidity resulting from the fast.
- Drink at least 2¹/₂ cups of this broth daily during the fast.

On rising the next day: drink either camomile or peppermint tea (unsweetened), a cup of vegetable broth, or a cup of half spring water and half carrot juice, beetroot juice, or warm or cold apple juice.

A selection of one of these items, or bottled spring water, should be consumed at 2- to 3-hourly intervals during the day, making sure that the vegetable broth is consumed at least twice during the day (not less than 2½ cups daily) and that the total liquid intake is not less than 10 cups and not more than 20 cups daily.

If you cannot obtain fresh vegetable juice, then bottled organic vegetable juice is available at most health food stores, suitable for use in fasting as long as it does not contain preservatives (other than lactic acid) and is guaranteed organically grown.

- Carrot and beetroot are the ideal juices.
- Continue this pattern for the 2 or 3 days of the fast.

Finish the fast by eating, on the evening of the final day, one of the following 'meals':

○ purée of cooked apple or pear, or
○ purée of carrot plus a little puréed vegetable soup, or
○ live natural yogurt.

Chew all food very thoroughly and slowly when breaking a fast.

The next morning eat yogurt and grated apple, or a fresh pear meal, and have a salad and baked potato for the lunch meal, continuing thereafter on a normal pattern of eating.

The advice for ending a fast depends upon a person not being sensitive to any of the foods mentioned. If dairy produce, for example, is in any way suspect then it should play no part in breaking a fast.

For this reason, anyone with suspected allergies should take advice or be under some degree of supervision during this time.

If necessary (in cases of chronic constipation or chronic allergy) an herbal laxative or castor oil could be used on the last evening of the fast, or a warm water enema may be used.

If the person who is fasting is chronically ill, then daily, small warm water enemas should be used during the fast. The hygiene of the bowel can be further improved by employing one or all of the following during the fast, and for a week or so afterwards:

○ Take daily: Half of a teaspoon of *Lactobacillus acidophilus* and half a teaspoon of *Bifidobacteria* culture (good health stores stock freeze-dried cultures of these friendly bacteria). These highly concentrated products will enhance the flora of the bowel.

○ *Note:* There are also versions which are suitable for people who are milk sensitive.

○ If bowel toxicity is a factor (chronic constipation, for example):

    ○ Stir 1 teaspoon of fine green clay powder (make sure it is a French source – obtainable from many health stores) into a small glass of spring water and allow it to settle, for an hour. Drink the water, but not the sediment. Do this at least once a day during the fast and for a week after. The clay has a detoxifying quality and soothes the bowel.

6: Immune Enhancement: Supplements, Herbs, Hydrotherapy, and Acupuncture

In this chapter we will look at tactics which can support immune enhancement by means of herbal medicines and nutritional supplements as well as dietary strategies. We are also going to examine evidence from research into the use of hydrotherapy – one involving extreme heat (hyperthermia) to deactivate invading microorganisms, and the other using regular cold showers or baths to enhance 'hardiness' and greater immune efficiency.

These methods can be used safely at home – if the guidelines given are followed.

In this chapter we will also consider the amazing immune-enhancing effects of acupuncture – a method which obviously calls for the help of a qualified practitioner.

Nutrition and Immune Function

Nutritional methods to enhance immune function can be divided into three essentially different but overlapping areas:

1 The need for a sound nutritional base to maintain your health and well-being.
2 Nutritional strategies which you can learn to use to enhance the way your immune system functions.

3 Nutritional strategies which can be used in specific circumstances to ease particular symptoms and conditions.

TO EACH HIS OWN

We are all different and it is certain that there is no universal dietary prescription which will suit everyone. In each of the three categories mentioned above, every one of us starts from a different place, with diverse histories in terms of health and diet, and unique biochemical requirements which are inborn.[1]

○ Some people will have eaten sensibly in the past (and in the present); others may be nutritionally deficient because of an unbalanced diet.
○ Some of us will be able to absorb nutrients from food efficiently; others may have a weakened digestive system and be unable to absorb easily the essential nutrients in food.
○ Some people will have accumulated toxic debris from past use of drugs, junk food, and exposure to pollutants; others will have no such burden.
○ As a result of what is known as 'biochemical individuality,' some people's specific nutrient requirements will differ vastly from others' – because of genetic factors over which they have no control.

This means that only general nutritional guidelines can be given as to ways in which immune function can be improved. The suggestions given here are not meant as a prescription for you to follow precisely; advice from a suitably qualified and licensed health care professional is necessary to provide responsible nutritional guidelines, taking into account what is unique about your particular needs.

Natural Alternatives to Antibiotics

GENERAL NUTRITIONAL GUIDELINES FOR IMMUNE ENHANCEMENT

When anyone has a weakened immune system it has been shown that malnutrition is one of the most significant factors, whatever else may be happening. How well nourished you are helps to decide how fast your health declines when the immune system has been weakened. Nutritional factors help decide how vulnerable and how susceptible you are to disease in general and infection in particular.[2]

Without good nutrition, all other therapeutic efforts are much less likely to succeed.

If you want to help your immune system, then the evidence is that a balanced wholefood diet (*see page 124*) is essential. This means that even a good balanced diet should be accompanied by specific supplementation, according to needs, to help immune efficiency.

The reasons why your nutritional status might be less than perfect can include:

- poor choice of what food you eat
- poor digestion and absorption of what you eat – even if it is balanced
- problems in the way whatever is digested and absorbed is actually handled in your body because of disturbed transportation and use of the nutrients.

There are just a few absolute 'rules' about what we should do in our eating habits, which are meant for everyone. There are also some universal and specific 'don'ts.'

The immune-enhancement 'rules' which you may want to take note of include:

- Refined carbohydrates (sugar of any color, white flour products, etc.) have been shown to depress immune function and should be avoided. We should eat these things in only small quantities and only now and then.[3]

○ Saturated fats and a high-fat diet make digestion less efficient. By increasing the levels of cholesterol and certain fats in the body, they also lead directly to a reduction in the efficiency of specific aspects of immune function (for example antibody production becomes less effective, response to infectious agents is weakened, etc.).[4] For this reason, animal fats in general should be avoided or reduced (meat and dairy products, for example), although oils from fish and many plants are helpful in promoting immune function and so can form a major part of your diet.[5]

○ Alcohol and caffeine, not surprisingly, have been shown to affect immune efficiency and should be excluded from the diet completely if you are already immune deficient, or reduced considerably if you want to keep your immune system healthy.[6]

○ If your digestive system is not easily able to handle raw foods such as vegetables, then eat them lightly cooked (steamed, stir-fried, in soups, stews, etc.) as this will help to break down the materials which your digestive system is having trouble with.

○ The amount of protein you eat needs to be kept at a high level in order to supply your body with the raw material for energy production and repair. Non-fat live yogurt, fish (especially cold-water varieties), free-range poultry and lean meat (game, for preference, as this has lower fat levels than domesticated animal sources) all offer easily digested protein.

○ If on the other hand you choose a vegetarian mode of eating, then you have to ensure a daily combination of pulses and grains or nuts/seeds (unless there is allergy/sensitivity to any of these), as these combine to provide your body with complete protein.

○ A daily supplement of the 'building blocks' of protein, free-form amino acids (powder or capsule) can guarantee a good, virtually predigested source of protein (*see supplement suggestions below*), can be very useful if weight loss is a goal, and helps when the immune system is weakened.

○ The amount of proteins compared with the amount of carbohydrates and fats which are eaten also seems to be important. This has been emphasized by a wide range of health experts. Suggestions are given later in this chapter.[7]

The next list made up the 'ten-point nutritional guidelines' issued to people taking part in the Bastyr College Healing AIDS Research Project (HARP) which was designed to enhance the immune function of severely immune-compromised individuals. We can learn a great deal to help our own immune systems from this.[8]

Immune-enhancement Guidelines

1 Eat whole food – as 'dense' as is manageable (containing essential nutrients and requiring chewing).
2 Organic and fresh vegetables, fruits and proteins (fish/meat) are best whenever they are available.
3 Reduce or eliminate simple sugars and replace with complex carbohydrates (vegetables, whole grains, bean family of foods, etc.) which are rich in nutrients (zinc, etc.).
4 Reduce polyunsaturated and saturated fats and oils.
5 Use monounsaturated instead (such as olive oil) with special emphasis on omega-3 oils (fish and certain plant oils such as flaxseed and evening primrose, for example).
6 Eat little and often throughout the day to improve absorption of nutrients from food.
7 Try to keep a balance of food intake which ensures 65 percent of what you eat is complex carbohydrates (vegetables, fruits, pulses, grains), 15 percent protein (fish, yogurt, eggs, meat), and 20 percent fat.
8 If you have a 'delicate' digestive system, make sure that the fruits and vegetables you eat are thoroughly clean and free of parasites and bacteria, and easier to digest, by steaming them lightly before eating.

9 Eat a wide variety of foods to help avoid becoming 'sensitized' to specific food families through frequent repetition.
10 Avoid altogether chocolate, caffeine, and alcohol if at all
possible.[9]

The following is a sample day's diet for anyone who is immune
compromised, or anyone who wants to make their immune
system work better:

Breakfast

Choose two or three selections from:

1 mixed seeds (sunflower, pumpkin, sesame, linseed) and grains
(wheat or oat or millet or rice flakes or whole grains). The seeds
can be eaten whole or milled. These can be lightly oven-roasted
or soaked overnight in a little water to soften them, and eaten on
their own or with live low-fat yogurt and fresh fruit.
2 oatmeal (or millet) porridge plus fresh almonds or walnuts
3 vegetable or fish soup – with whole rice or noodles if preferred
4 live low-fat yogurt or kefir (a fermented milk drink)
5 sourdough rye or wheat bread or toast (depending on sensitivi-
ties/allergies) with olive oil or cottage cheese (low fat) or egg
(see point 8 below)
6 enzyme-rich fruit such as papaya
7 tofu (bean curd) stir-fried with vegetables
8 two or three eggs weekly (boiled, poached, scrambled)
9 herbal teas or spring water to drink.

Mid-morning and Mid-afternoon Snacks

1 rice cakes or any of the items listed under 'breakfast'.

1   unless you have chosen a vegetarian diet, at least one of these meals should contain an animal protein source such as fish, free-range poultry (avoiding skin) or game (to avoid antibiotics and steroids given to most farm-reared animals). If fish is chosen then a cold-water type such as herring, salmon, sardine, haddock, sole, or cod is better because of the types of useful oils they contain. Cook by boiling, steaming, grilling, baking, stir-frying, poaching (try to avoid frying or roasting, as this alters the nature of any fat content) or use the fish, poultry, or meat in a soup. For the best digestive efficiency, protein should be eaten with green vegetables and/or seaweed lightly cooked in one of the ways mentioned above. Seasoning should be by use of herbs (garlic) and spices with as little salt as possible (or you can use seasoning such as miso). If any oil is used in cooking it should be virgin olive oil (or sunflower oil) which can also be used as a dressing.

2   the other main meal should be similar or could be based on a combination of pulses (chickpeas, mung beans, lentils, kidney or any other sort of bean) and grains (millet, brown rice, quinoa, amaranth, buckwheat, etc. – whole or as pasta/noodles). A soup, stew, roast or other combination of these ingredients (pulses/grains) provides your body with a first-class source of protein. Low-fat cheese (cottage cheese, for example) or tofu can also be eaten as a good source of protein. A variety of starchy vegetables (lightly cooked) such as carrots, beets, squash, potatoes as well as green vegetables are also highly desirable. There is abundant evidence of the health-enhancing value of brassica vegetables (cabbage, kale, broccoli). If your digestion is sound, include raw salad vegetables as well.

3   desserts should be low-fat yogurt (live) or enzyme-rich fruit (papaya, apple, pear).

Note

This brief 'menu' is not definitive but gives you an idea of a framework in which 4 or 5 snack meals daily are consumed, providing ample basic nutrition.

In almost all cases where a weakened immune system exists, additional nutrient (supplement) support is helpful and desirable – if financially possible.

NUTRITIONAL SUPPORT FOR IMMUNE FUNCTION

Note

Many of the references for this information derive from research into the most obvious immune-deficiency situation – people with AIDS. We can all learn a lot about immune function from this research. Even if you only have mild immune deficiency (frequent colds and flu, for example) this knowledge can still be helpful. Malnutrition is common in people who have weakened immune systems.[10]

○ Swallowing supplements or having nutrients injected (intramuscular or intravenous methods may be used if the condition is serious, as appropriate) are the only ways of ensuring that adequate nutrients get into the body. If you have a weakened digestive system, taking supplements orally does not guarantee that they will arrive where they are needed.
○ A number of herbal medicines have been shown to have very beneficial effects on digestion, absorption and on aspects of immune function. These will be outlined below.
○ If you are trying to improve immune function nutritionally, the taking of supplements can usually be safely combined with herbal methods (along with methods which also bring into play the immune-modulating power of the mind, as discussed in Chapter 5).

Proven Deficiencies

The following are a few of the known deficiencies associated with most people who have weakened immune function:[11]

Vitamin B$_6$[12]
Folate[13]
Vitamin B$_{12}$[14]
Selenium[15]
Zinc[16]

Nutritional supplementation has been shown in research studies to offer great benefits to people already seriously ill with immune deficiency, and is seen by many to be a cornerstone of improving immune system function.[17]

In one study which lasted six months, vitamins, minerals, amino acids, and essential fatty acids were all supplemented. Among the benefits which were seen were a general improvement in well-being and a significant gain in important aspects of immune function.

In the following list, dosage ranges are given which are commonly advised for people with severe immune deficiency. *These recommendations should not be seen as suggestions for self-treatment.* Ideally you should get advice from a suitably qualified health care professional before taking high-dosage nutrient supplements. In some instances, such as high-dosage beta-carotene (which your body turns into vitamin A) and/or vitamin C and/or zinc supplementation (for example) the nutrient is not only replacing possible deficiencies but may be acting in a 'pharmacological' way – that is, it may actually inhibit or kill bacteria, viruses, or fungi.

It is important not to exceed the recommended dose, as some nutrients can be toxic in high doses (as can anything else, including water and oxygen!). This applies in particular to fat-soluble nutrients such as vitamins A and E as well as to minerals such as selenium and zinc, and to the B-vitamin pyridoxine (B$_6$). Stay inside the guideline recommendations to be safe, and if at all possible get responsible advice about your particular needs.

Multi-vitamin/mineral Supplement

As an 'insurance' against deficiency and in place of a number of the individual nutrients listed below, a soundly constructed multi-vitamin/mineral supplement is suggested in order to provide an underlying source of nutrients. There are, however, no multi-vitamin/mineral formulations with sufficiently high dosages to meet the needs required when immune function is low.

An antioxidant formulation which contains vitamins A, C, E and (usually) the minerals selenium and/or zinc can be taken to replace the individual antioxidant ingredients as listed below – but only if the formulation is sufficiently well constructed so that potency/dosage of the nutrients are adequate.

Pro-vitamin A (Beta-carotene)

A dose of between 100,000 and 300,000 iu of beta-carotene is used in treating active immune-deficiency conditions. This form of vitamin A is basically non-toxic (unlike vitamin A itself, which should only be taken in small amounts unless you are under expert guidance). Beta-carotene is a powerful free radical scavenger (antioxidant) and this is important in reducing viral damage. It is also capable of actually killing some disease-causing viruses.[18,19] 300,000 iu per day will have antiviral effects, protect against tissue damage and raise levels of specific immune-enhancing lymphocytes. When supplemented (in doses of 100,000 to 200,000 iu daily) it improves helper T-cell levels in healthy individuals as well as in those with immune depression. If excess amounts are being taken your skin may take on an orange tinge (resembling a slight sunburn). This is completely harmless and will fade when doses are reduced.[20]

Vitamin C (Ascorbic Acid)

Vitamin C is a powerful antioxidant and has been shown to be able to control many viruses and bacteria as well as having specific and potent immune-enhancing effects.[21,22,23]

High-dose use of vitamin C has been shown to act against bacteria and viral activity in general as well as to protect tissues against inflammatory damage resulting from bacteria and virus activity. Vitamin C has specific antiviral activity (particularly against what are known as retroviruses) and boosts immune function, specifically of macrophages and neutrophils.[24,25,26,27]

During active infection dosage is sometimes suggested in terms of 'according to bowel tolerance.' This means stepping up the intake of vitamin C, day by day – by between 500 mg to 1 gram per day – until diarrhea develops. At this time the dose is reduced to that taken the previous day and maintained at this level (as long as no diarrhea develops, in which case the dosage must be reduced again). Because of our unique biochemical individuality some people reach bowel tolerance when taking as little as 3 to 4 grams a day, whereas someone else may have to take much more before bowel looseness occurs.[28] (It should be noted that a recent study has found that between 1 gram and 5 grams of Vitamin C daily may cause gene changes.)

Calcium, sodium or magnesium ascorbate (forms of vitamin C) are all easily available; magnesium ascorbate is considered by many to be a superior form for the body to use.[29] Even when vitamin C is supplemented in very modest doses (just 200 mg daily) by apparently healthy elderly individuals there is a marked improvement in immune function.

Vitamin E

Vitamin E is also a powerful antioxidant and protects the integrity of your cell walls.

Doses of between 400 and 800 iu daily are usually suggested when someone is being treated for an illness, however just 200 iu daily is recommended for protection and maintenance. The production of antibodies is increased when Vitamin E is supplemented, especially when accompanied by the mineral selenium. Deficiency of vitamin E and/or selenium leads to a decline in T and B cells.[30]

Selenium

This mineral works in cooperation with vitamin E and is a vital constituent of important enzymes such as glutathione peroxidase, which protects cell wall integrity (remember that to infect you, bacteria and viruses commonly attack the cell wall). 200 micrograms of selenium daily should be supplemented in the case of immune deficiency. When healthy individuals who are attempting to enhance immune function took this amount daily for 8 weeks, they produced over 100 percent increase in lymphocyte activity.[31,32]

Zinc

Practically all people with a weakened immune system are also deficient in a range of important mineral nutrients, with zinc being one of the most important of these.[33,34] Nearly 100 important enzymes depend upon adequate presence of zinc, and many of these are involved in immune function. Tests can prove whether or not there is a deficiency although just a look at a person's range of symptoms can suggest zinc is probably deficient. Among these are: skin lesions (ulceration, thickening, dryness), loss of hair, loss of appetite and reduced sense of smell, lethargy, and increased susceptibility to infection. When apparently healthy men were supplemented with zinc (150 mg daily) for 4 weeks their T-cell function increased markedly.

If excessive amounts of zinc are supplemented this can depress immune function, so it is important to take the amounts suggested. Supplementation with 30 to 50 mg daily is usual for maintenance, with higher doses (double those listed) for a week or so during an infection.

Potassium and Magnesium

Potassium is commonly deficient in people with immune depression. You can make sure of enough potassium by eating a diet rich in vegetables.

Natural Alternatives to Antibiotics

Magnesium is commonly deficient in Western diets and especially so in people with immune depression. Supplementation of 500 mg daily is usually suggested by nutritionists.

Iron and Manganese

Iron is commonly deficient when there is immune depression, but should be supplemented only under expert guidance.

Manganese is an important but neglected mineral involved in many enzyme processes. Deficiency is common. 5 to 10 mg daily is usually recommended; this amount will often be found in a multi-vitamin/mineral formulation.

Essential Fatty Acids

Omega 3 and Omega 6 fatty acids such as linolenic acid and gamma linolenic acid are essential (which means that the body cannot manufacture them and has to have them provided in the diet). Their importance in malabsorption problems and immune dysfunction is now well understood, as is their ability to help control inflammation. Linolenic acid and gamma linolenic acid (GLA) derived from the Evening Primrose plant, Blackcurrant seeds, Borage (herb) or Linseed as well as from fish oils (which provide eicosapentenoic acid – EPA) are suggested for anyone with a compromised digestive and/or immune system – dosage of between 1 and 3 grams daily is a common recommendation.[35]

Probiotics

Almost every person with immune system problems has a compromised internal ecology affecting their bowel flora. When the flora are healthy they help to detoxify the bowel, manufacture B vitamins and keep yeasts and undesirable bacteria in check. As we have seen, the flora are easily damaged by antibiotics, steroid drugs, unbalanced diet, and stress. Repopulation ('reflorastation') of the intestines requires two organisms in particular to be regularly supplemented: *L. acidophilus* (for the small intestine) and *Bifidobacteria* (for the colon). This is especially urgent if yeasts (such as Candida albicans) are present and active. Dosage depends on the strain which you are taking – expert advice is urged. Guidelines are given in Chapter 9 as to how to use these friendly bacteria if antibiotics are being or have been used.[36]

Vitamin B-complex

One or two slow-release B-complex capsules are commonly suggested to be taken daily, formulated to a high potency (50 to 100 mg of each of the major B vitamins – some of which may also be taken individually, depending upon your particular needs).[37]

Note

Yeast-free sources of B vitamins are recommended by many experts to avoid possible aggravation of sensitivities resulting from yeast infections such as Candida albicans (*see Chapter 7*).

Individual B vitamins may sometimes be recommended by a nutritional expert, however more usually the entire complex of associated B-vitamins would be taken together. If single B-vitamins are recommended, it is important also to supplement with B-complex to avoid imbalances which single-nutrient supplementation may cause.

The B vitamins which clearly influence immune function include the following:

○ Thiamin (B_1) – produces a decline in immune function when deficient
○ Riboflavin (B_2) – required for antibody production.
Deficiency leads to decline in T and B cells. It is partially manufactured by a healthy bowel flora.

O Pyridoxine (B_6) – needed for antibody production. Deficiency leads to T-cell decline and reduction in the size of the thymus gland. Remember that excess (over 200 mg daily) is potentially toxic if supplementation is prolonged.

O Pantothenic acid (B_5) – involved in altered T- and B-cell ratios when deficient (*see Chapter 5*). Viral infection is also more common when B_5 is in short supply.

O Vitamin B_{12} – another key player in T- and B-cell efficiency. Supplementation is essential if digestive function is impaired.

O Folic acid – very important in any attempts at improving weakened immune function. Resistance to infection is poor when this is deficient.[38]

O Biotin – a B-vitamin usually produced by a healthy bowel flora. It becomes deficient as a result of damage to the 'friendly bacteria' of the intestines (often after excessive antibiotic usage) and its absence, or deficiency, is thought to allow yeast to turn from a simple to an aggressive, invasive form. For this reason it is often supplemented as part of an anti-Candida program.[39]

Herbs to Help Immune Function

Use of herbal medicine in treating a compromised immune system is well researched. It has also attracted the attention of major pharmaceutical manufacturers, since if they can slightly modify a natural product and patent this, a bonanza awaits their shareholders.

The following list of herbal substances comprises a representation of the best and brightest examples of what is available, and of some of their major uses. This is not a recommendation to use them, as your particular needs may be special. Try to take advice before using herbs for health problems, except for the short term to help with simple conditions.

Allium Sativum (Garlic)

This is a powerful antibacterial, antiviral, antiparasitic, and anti-fungal agent. There is recent evidence of anti-HIV potential.[40] It is also effective against worms and protozoa, including organisms resistant to standard antibiotics.[41,42,43]

Garlic has been used for thousands of years as a food and a medicine, and is currently attracting enormous research interest because of its safety and efficacy. The active ingredient of garlic, which has the antibiotic effects, is allicin – which also carries the most obvious indication of its use – the smell. Fortunately methods have been found to develop garlic with all its potency intact yet without the odor!

Astragalus membranaceus

This has long been used to enhance immune function in Chinese medicine. It produces increased phagocytosis (the 'eating' of invading bacteria by immune system cells), enhanced T-cell transformation, increased numbers of macrophages and increased IgA and IgG levels, while inducing the formation of interferon (a protein substance produced by virus-invaded cells that prevents reproduction of the virus) and enhancing blastogenesis (the formation of new cells) in the white blood cells of normal and cancer patients.[44,45]

Dionaea muscipula –Venus FlyTrap Plant (Carnivora)

This is an immune stimulator and modulator. It increases the number and activity of T-cells and increases the phagocytosis of macrophages. It is used intravenously, intramuscularly, by inhalation and orally.[46,47,48]

Echinacea angustifolia (and E. purpurea)

This is an amazingly useful and safe herb which has powerful immune-enhancing properties including macrophage activation, as well as inhibiting viral, fungal and bacterial infections.

The effect of Echinacea seems to be directly on the thymus gland, which as we have seen is a vital component of immune defense.

Extracts of the root of Echinacea have been shown in research to include substances such as inulin, which activates the production of a wide range of immune chemicals.

Echinacea has been a traditional Native American herbal substance for centuries, and has now been widely researched and used throughout the world. It can be taken in capsule form or as a liquid (as an alcohol extract). Many experts believe this (liquid) form to be superior in that it is absorbed and used by the body more efficiently. Liquid extract of Echinacea, taken by healthy individuals (30 drops 3 times a day for 5 days) boosts the presence of leucocytes (white blood cells) by around 40 percent. When used by people with infection it acts in numerous ways, boosting defenses as well as acting directly on bacterial cell membranes to make them more vulnerable.[49,50]

A dose of 3 to 4 500-mg capsules at least twice daily is usually suggested during an infection. Combination capsules and liquids are now available in which Echinacea and other herbs are combined for a potent effect against infection and to enhance immune function.

Ginseng (or Eleutherococcus – 'Siberian Ginseng')

These are adaptogens, which help your body withstand the harmful effects of all forms of stress and which also have tonic effects on the thymus gland – vital for the production of T-cells (*see Chapter 7*).[51,52]

Glycyrrhiza Glabra (Licorice)

This immune system-enhancer[53] improves macrophage activity and increases the production of interferon. Licorice extract also has broad-spectrum antimicrobial effects.[54]

In addition it is an antioxidant, protecting tissues, especially those in the liver, from free radical damage.[55]

Glycyrrhizin is also an anti-inflammatory agent and protects against allergy and its effects, most notably those related to skin conditions.[56,57]

It seems to protect the thymus gland from shrinking when steroids such as cortisone are used, and actually enhances the anti-inflammatory effects of cortisone.[58]

As far as immune support is concerned, this remarkable herb acts against numerous undesirable pathogenic bacteria (*Staphylococcus aureus*, for example, and Candida albicans). For many naturopathic and herbal practitioners, this is the herb of first choice in dealing with viral infections (three 500-mg capsules 4 times daily during infection).[59,60,61]

Hydrastis canandensis (Goldenseal)

This is an immune enhancer involved in macrophage activation, increasing natural killer cell activity and enhancing gastrointestinal function (it is particularly effective against diarrhea). It is antibacterial, antifungal, anti-yeast (Candida albicans). For many naturopathic and herbal practitioners this is the first choice for use in treating bacterial infection (four 500-mg capsules four times daily during infection).[62,63,64]

Hypericum perforatum (St. John's Wort)

This is commonly used for its antibacterial and antiviral qualities. In doses of around 1,500 mg daily (in divided doses) it enhances the function of the immune system – apparently by improving circulation to the spleen – increasing macrophage activity.[65,66,67]

There is recent strong German research evidence of Hypericum's usefulness in combating moderate depression – something which therefore also helps reduce the harmful effect of depression on immune function.

Isatis

This is a broad-spectrum antibacterial, antiviral herb which calms inflammation and lowers temperature.[68]

Melaleuca alternifolia (Tea Tree Oil)

This versatile Australian oil can be used on the surface of the body or diluted as a gargle or douche to treat most fungal and many bacterial infections. Caution should be used in applying it neat as it can irritate the skin.

Laboratory studies by Giles Elsom of the University of East London have shown that Tea Tree Oil is effective against antibiotic-resistant bacteria including *Staphylococcus aureus* (Methicillin-resistant Staph. aureus – MRSA). He says, 'Tea tree oil is safer than antibiotics and it is non-toxic. In the long term our aim would be to wash people as they enter wards to stop them bringing in infection.'[69]

Usnea barbata

The extract of this European 'plant' (a lichen – so really more of a cross between a fungus and an algae) has powerful antibiotic effects on some of the nastiest bacterial agents – including *Staphylococcus* spp and *Mycobacterium tuberculosis*. It is taken as a liquid extract, starting (to ensure tolerance) with 3 to 4 drops in water twice a day and building up to around 10 drops 3 times a day during an active infection. It can also be used for sore throats as a gargle (1 drop in enough water to gargle with), and as a douche for vaginal infections. Ideally it should be used under expert guidance as it can irritate the stomach and bowels if used excessively. Some experts claim that it is a more powerful antibacterial agent than penicillin, but far safer.[70]

There are many studies quoted in Werbach and Murray's *Botanical Influences on Illness* (Tarzana, CA: Third Line Press, 1995) which indicate the value of herbal products such as:

○ garlic (which inhibits viral, bacterial, fungal, protozoal and parasitic infections)
○ echinacea (for skin, upper respiratory, antiviral, antifungal and antibacterial effects)
○ bromelaine (for sinusitis, urinary tract infections, enhancement of the effectiveness of antibiotics)
○ Berberine (for treatment of Coxsackie-B virus, trachoma, giardia, *Entamoeba hystolytica*, etc.)
○ pollen extracts – have been shown to reduce the severity of upper respiratory infections which are common in competitive swimmers. During 6 weeks of supplementation, those receiving pollen had only 4 days of illness as opposed to 27 days in those patients who were given a dummy (placebo) medication.[71]

Note
All herbal compounds and many individual herbs are toxic if used in excessive amounts. Many produce mild digestive side-effects.[72] Advice from an expert is always prudent.

Hydrotherapy

It may surprise you to know that hydrotherapy can be used to treat viral and bacterial infection or to enhance immune function.

There are two contrasting approaches to immune enhancement and treatment of infection using water therapies:

1 The use of heat to increase core body temperature and so create an 'artificial fever.'
2 The use of cold showers, cold baths, or alternating cold and hot wet compresses, to enhance immune function.

Both approaches have been researched and both can be adapted for home use.

1/ HYPERTHERMIA (ARTIFICIAL FEVER THERAPY)

Fever is one of the body's most powerful defenses against disease. Hyperthermia artificially induces fever in the patient who is unable to mount a natural fever response to infection, inflammation or other health challenges. It is used locally or over the entire body to treat diseases ranging from viral infections to cancer, and is an effective self-help treatment for colds and flus.

Viruses and bacteria are heat-sensitive; some more so than others (as are cancer cells) – and for this reason a number of different methods of heating the body have been used to encourage the deactivation or death of viruses, bacteria, and cancer cells.[73]

Recently, medical research has begun to examine these methods more extensively.[74] In some clinic settings, most notably in Germany, up to 8 hours of immersion in hot water (with frequent cool drinks and cool compresses on the head/neck) is used. This is extremely tiring for the patient, and less exhausting methods are suggested, especially for home use (but still under some sort of supervision or guidance).

In a research study conducted at Bastyr University, Seattle in 1990, participants with HIV infection were given a series of 12 hyperthermia baths (38.8°C/102°F) for 40 minutes. These were given twice weekly for three weeks at a time, over the course of a year.

Some clinics use hyperthermic baths at far higher temperatures than this (50°C/122°F and more), although there is some evidence that brain damage can occur at such very high temperatures.[75]

For safety, therefore, the heat levels suggested by the Bastyr College HARP (Healing AIDS Research Project) study are thought best, unless the person undergoing the hyperthermia is under constant expert supervision.[76,77]

How Hyperthermia Works

A state of hyperthermia exists when body temperature increases above its normal level of 37°C (98.6°F). An increase in body temperature causes many useful defensive physiological responses to occur in the body. Hyperthermia takes advantage of the fact that many invading organisms tolerate a narrower temperature range than do our body tissues, and are therefore more susceptible to increases in temperature. They may die from overheating before harm is done to human tissue. Examples are viruses such as rhinovirus[78] (responsible for one half of all respiratory infections), HIV,[79] and the microorganisms and bacteria that cause syphilis and gonorrhea.[80]

Hyperthermia treatment may not be able to kill every invading organism, but can reduce their numbers to a level the immune system can more easily handle. Hyperthermia stimulates the immune system by increasing the production of antibodies and interferon (produced by virus-invaded cells and preventing reproduction of the virus). Hyperthermia is also useful in detoxification therapy because it releases, and encourages elimination from the body of, toxins stored in fat cells.

Methods of Inducing Hyperthermia

Body temperature can be increased swiftly by applying heat externally. This approach causes engorgement of the small blood vessels near the surface of the skin and starts the body perspiring in an attempt to control the increase in temperature.

An increase in body temperature may be accomplished by such low-tech methods as immersing the body in hot water, sitting in a sauna or steam bath, or wrapping yourself in blankets with a hot water bottle. Other, more 'high-tech' approaches more commonly found in hospitals and medical centers include the use of shortwave or microwave diathermy (heat treatment), ultrasound, radiant heating, and extra-corporeal heating (heat generated outside the body, by machine, a compress or in any other way).

Hyperthermia can be produced either locally or over the whole body. Locally applied hyperthermia is most often employed to treat infections such as upper respiratory illness (by inhaling steam or using diathermy on the area), or for infected wounds of the hand or foot (immersing the injured part in hot water). Whole-body hyperthermia, on the other hand, is used where there is a general infection, where a local application is impractical, or where a general whole-body response is desirable.

Viral Infection and Hyperthermic Therapy

At the Natural Health Clinic of Bastyr University, hyperthermia is commonly used in the treatment of HIV and other chronic and acute viral infections. In 1988 and 1989, Bastyr's Healing AIDS Research Project (HARP) included hyperthermia in the treatment protocol developed for the study because of its immune-stimulating, detoxifying, and disinfecting properties.

According to Leanna Standish, Ph.D., N.D., when HARP participants were asked to describe what aspect of treatment had the greatest impact, they chorused 'hyperthermia.' There was a decrease in night sweats and in the frequency of secondary infection. Also, many participants reported having a greater sense of well-being after hyperthermia.[81]

Laboratory research has proven that the HIV virus is temperature-sensitive and suffers progressively greater inactivation at temperatures above 37°C (98.6°F). After 30 minutes' heating in a water bath at 42°C (107.6°F), 40 percent inactivation of HIV virus has been reported, and at 56°C (132.8°F), 100 percent inactivation results.[82]

'I don't believe that hyperthermia is the answer for all HIV patients,' says Dr Doug Lewis, Director of the Natural Health Clinic, 'but I do think it is an appropriate adjunct treatment for all but a few very sick patients.'

Risks Associated with Hyperthermia

When used knowledgeably and with care, hyperthermia is a safe and effective treatment for many conditions. Ill-effects of hyperthermia usually appear only when body temperatures exceed 41°C (106°F). However, certain individuals are more sensitive to the effects of heat and their conditions should be treated with great care. These include people with anemia, heart disease, diabetes, seizure disorders, and tuberculosis.

Other reported risks of hyperthermia include herpes outbreaks[83] (including herpes zoster), liver toxicity,[84] and nervous system injury. Hyperthermia for detoxification should only be done under medical supervision for the reasons described.

Hyperthermia at Home

Hot baths are the simplest method of inducing a fever at home and can be used to treat upper respiratory tract infections (colds, flu) and even lower respiratory tract problems such as bronchitis and pneumonia.

To treat viral infections, hot baths can be combined with hot drinks and blanket wrapping to stimulate the immune system. After a hot bath, wrap yourself in dry blankets. You may also want to put a hot water bottle over your abdomen. Allow yourself to perspire heavily for as long as you can tolerate this. It may take several hours. Follow with a cool shower.

It is also possible to produce a mild fever at home simply by wrapping up in a dry blanket pack. Again, you can allow yourself to perspire heavily for several hours and follow with a cool shower.

A wet sheet pack may also be used to produce a fever. Here you wrap in a very cold, wet (just damp – not dripping wet) sheet and several blankets. As with the dry pack, you will need several hours to produce a fever. The cold sheet produces reactions in the body that encourage the production of heat. It is often useful first to heat yourself up by exercising or having a hot bath or shower before using the wet sheet pack.

Local hyperthermia can also be useful at times. One study shows that the inhalation of steam is useful in the treatment of head colds.[85] Hot packs or hot soaks may also be used to treat local conditions. An infection in the hand or foot might benefit from being immersed in hot water. A local infection that will not allow for full immersion might be treated with hot packs applied to the area.

2/ HYDROTHERAPY TO ENHANCE IMMUNE FUNCTION

The results of important hydrotherapy research in London involving 100 volunteers were published in *The European* newspaper on 22nd and 29th April, 1993. The Thrombosis Research Institute (which conducted the research) claims that the use of this form of self-treatment proves without question the value of carefully graduated cold baths, regularly taken (six months' daily use is suggested for optimal results).

The Institute, under its director Dr. Vijay Kakkar, have now gathered 5,000 volunteers for the next stage of this research into the benefits of what has been called Thermo Regulatory Hydrotherapy (TRH).

The results of the first study showed that, when applied correctly, TRH has a number of beneficial effects, including:

- very much enhanced levels of white blood cells – the body's first-line defenders against infection
- a boost to sex hormone production, which influences potency in men and fertility in women
- renewed energy: many sufferers from chronic fatigue syndrome were found to improve dramatically
- improved circulation in people with cold extremities. Circulation is found to improve rapidly with TRH.
- reduced incidence of heart attack and stroke, as a result of improved blood-clotting function
- reduced levels of unpleasant menopausal symptoms.

This research involved taking graduated cold baths (*see 'The Method of TRH', below*) and closely mirrored previous research conducted in 1990 at Hanover Medical School in Germany. In this German study, students were asked to take either warm morning showers or cold ones. The level and intensity of infections (mainly colds) they suffered over the following six months were monitored. Those taking cold showers were asked to increase gradually the degree of coldness, so that by the end of the first three weeks they were taking a 2- to 3-minute shower with the water as cold as possible (if any of them developed a cold during the six-month trial they were told to stop taking cold showers for the duration of the illness and for one week afterwards).

By the end of the six-month trial those students taking cold showers had had half the number of colds compared with the group taking warm showers, and the colds they did have lasted half as long – they were less acute, and these students' immune systems cleared them up faster.

This trial gives clear evidence that regular cold showers offer an increase in resistance to infection as well as enhanced efficiency of the immune function should infection occur.[86]

Cold Shower Method

The cold shower method calls for observing the following guidelines:

○ Start with a cool to tepid shower (perhaps at body heat) and finish, after 2 minutes, with the water cooler than body heat.
○ Over the next three weeks, slowly increase the degree of coldness so that by the end of the third week the water is as it comes from the cold faucet.
○ Have a 2- to 3-minute cold shower every morning unless you actually have an infection, in which case stop until it is better and for one week after this.

Natural Alternatives to Antibiotics

○ After the cold shower, dry yourself thoroughly and dress warmly.
○ Ensure that the bathroom in which the shower is being taken is not cold, and that there are no drafts.

The Method of TRH Bathing

The other approach, as described in the Thrombosis Research report, involves four stages. To be successful it is thought that it is essential to 'train' the body toward the beneficial response by going through each of these stages in turn.

○ Equipment needed: a bath, a bath thermometer, a watch and a bath mat
○ The bathroom needs to be at a reasonably comfortable temperature – not too cold and not very hot.
○ The temperature of the water should eventually be as it comes from the faucet – cold – however it is possible to train toward the cold bath by first having a tepid bath for a few weeks, gradually making the water colder so that it goes below body heat, until having a really cold bath is no longer a shock.
○ The timing described below can also be modified so that at first the whole process takes just a few minutes as the various stages of immersion are passed through, with a slow increase in the timing of each stage as well as a reduction in temperature.

Note

When cold water treatments are used in people with chronic health problems, the degree of stimulus used (how cold the water is, and how long a time is spent immersed) needs to be modified so that a very SLOW increment in contrast is achieved, gradually training and 'hardening' the body to what is potentially a stress factor. The TRH program runs for 80 days, with the degree of coldness and the length of time in the water increased only gradually.

To plunge someone who is extremely fragile in their ability to handle stress of any sort into cold water straight from the faucet would be foolhardy, whereas taking a shower or bath in 'neutral' (body heat) water for a week before – extremely gradually – starting the process of, day by day, getting the water cooler and cooler, perhaps over a period of months before faucet-cold water is used, is both sensible and effective.

Stage 1
Stand in the bath in cold water (the range recommended is between 12.7°C and 18.3°C [59° and 65°F], but take account of the Note above as to how cold the water should be in relation to the degree of the subject's fragility/robustness) for between 1 and 5 minutes once fully used to the process, perhaps after some weeks, as the internal thermostat (in the hypothalamus portion of the brain) responds.

Have a non-slip mat in place and avoid standing still but 'walk' up and down the bath or march on the spot.

Stage 2
When fully used to the standing-in-cold-water process, perhaps after some weeks, the internal thermostat is now primed. At this stage, after standing for several minutes, sit down in the cold water for another 1 to 5 minutes (ideally the water should be up to the waist – so that the pooled blood in the lower half of the body is cooled, further influencing the hypothalamus and helping to decongest the pelvis).

Stage 3
After another 2 or 3 weeks when the daily immersion involves first standing, then sitting, we come to the most important part of the program, in which it is necessary to immerse the entire body up to the neck and back of the head in cold water. After first standing, then sitting, lie down in the water so that just the

face and head are clear. Gently and slowly move the arms and legs to ensure that the slightly warmer water touching the skin is not static, and the cooling effect continues. This stage ultimately lasts between 10 and 20 minutes, but could be for as little as 2 minutes at first, with the degree of coldness being adjusted according to sensitivity.

Stage 4

This is for 'rewarming.' Get out of the bath, towel dry, and move around for a few minutes. As warming takes place a pleasant glowing sensation will be felt in various precise locations such as the chest, feet, and between the shoulder blades.

The whole sequence, modified by reducing the time and temperature at first, needs to be done daily if the 'training' or 'hardening' effect is to be achieved. Some people find that several cold baths daily improve their energy and ability to function.

Contraindications

This cold water bath method is not recommended for people with well-established heart disease, high blood pressure, or chronic diseases that require regular prescription medication – unless a doctor has been consulted as to the use of TRH.

As time passes the water should be progressively colder, so that after some months of applying this method no warm water at all is used, only the water from the cold faucet. If the process is uncomfortable at first, shorten the exposure time in the water and make it less cold, as explained in the cold shower method discussed above.

CONSTITUTIONAL HYDROTHERAPY – WHOLE-BODY CIRCULATION ENHANCEMENT

Another approach to 'whole-body' circulation enhancement which has beneficial effects on immune function is called simply Constitutional Hydrotherapy and was devised by

American Naturopaths early in the 20th century as a method of health enhancement. This cannot be self-applied and requires someone to assist. The whole procedure takes around 25 minutes and should be conducted 3 times a week for at least a month to achieve benefits. It can be undertaken more frequently without harm (there are no risks or contraindications) and can be performed indefinitely as long as benefits are felt.

Constitutional Hydrotherapy (CH) – Home Application

○ Effects: CH has a non-specific 'balancing' effect, reducing chronic pain, enhancing immune function, boosting circulatory efficiency, and promoting healing. There are no contraindications since the degree of temperature contrast can be modified to take account of any degree of sensitivity, frailty, etc.
○ Materials:
  ○ somewhere to lie down
  ○ a full-sized sheet folded in two, or two single sheets
  ○ 1 blanket (wool if possible)
  ○ 2 bath towels (when folded in two, each should be able to reach from side to side and from shoulders to hips)
  ○ 2 hand towels (each should, as a single layer, be the same size as one of the larger towels folded in two)
  ○ hot and cold water

Please note again, *this method cannot be self-applied; help is needed.*

Method

1 The person to be treated undresses and lies down, face up, between the sheets and under one of the blankets.
2 Immerse the two bath towels in hot water and wring them out. Turn back the blanket and top sheet and place the hot towels, folded (to make 4 layers) onto the person's

trunk, so that they cover the person from side to side and from shoulders to hips.

3 Cover with the sheet and blanket and leave for 5 minutes.

4 Rinse one of the single-layer (small) towels in cold water, the other in hot. Wring out.

5 Turn back the blanket and top sheet. Place the 'new' (small) hot towel on top of the 'old' (large) hot towels and 'flip' so that the small hot towel is directly on the skin. Remove the old towels. Immediately place the small cold towel onto the small hot towel and flip again, so that the cold one is against the skin. Remove the small hot towel.

6 Cover with the sheet and leave for 10 minutes or until the cold towel is warmed.

7 Remove the previously cold (now warmed by body heat) towel. The person being treated should now turn over onto his or her stomach.

8 Repeat steps 2 to 6 for the back.

Notes

○ If using a bed, take precautions (such as plastic sheeting) not to get this wet.

○ 'Hot' water in this context is of a temperature high enough to prevent you leaving your hand in it for more than 5 seconds.

○ The coldest water from a running faucet is adequate for the 'cold' towel. If it is a hot summer's day, adding ice to the water is acceptable, so long as the resulting temperature contrast is acceptable to the patient.

○ If the person being treated feels cold after the cold towel is placed on him or her, use back, foot or hand massage – through the blanket and towel – or use visualization: ask the person being treated to think of a sunny beach, for example.

○ Most importantly, varying the differential between hot and cold – a slight difference for someone whose immune function and overall degree of vulnerability is poor, a greater contrast (very hot and very cold) for someone whose constitution is robust – allows for this method to be used on anyone at all.

Acupuncture to Enhance Immune Function

Acupuncture is often used along with other methods (herbal medicines, etc.) to improve immune function.

Preliminary studies at the Quan Yin Clinic in San Francisco show acupuncture to be beneficial in increasing a variety of immune functions, including:

○ white blood cell function and efficiency
○ T-cell production

as well as alleviating many of the symptoms relating to immune depression.

A TYPICAL ACUPUNCTURE TREATMENT

First-time patients generally fill out a questionnaire about their medical history. Following that they are interviewed by an acupuncturist. The practitioner will look carefully at the patient, observing the color of the face and the tongue's coating, taking note of the person's body language and tone of voice, and asking questions about eating and sleeping habits, emotional stress, etc. Finally, the practitioner will feel the wrist, testing the quality and strength of 12 different pulses which are used in Chinese medical diagnosis.

Needles may then be placed in any one of several points chosen from over 300 special sites. Traditional Chinese Medicine suggests that no more than 10 to 12 needles be used per treatment. In fact, the more experienced the acupuncturist, the fewer needles he or she will need to use.

Essentially, acupuncture is painless. Although you may experience a slight prickling sensation when the needles are inserted, a competent acupuncturist will not hurt you when placing the needles. You may feel a slight tugging or aching sensation that passes quickly.

To protect both the acupuncturist and patients from AIDS or hepatitis, all acupuncturists now use pre-sterilized, disposable needles.

Most treatments last approximately 45 minutes.

RESULTS

Outstanding general results have been obtained using acupuncture to treat immune-related problems, and in modifying many of the patient's symptoms.

Dr. William Michael Cargile, DC, L.Ac. has worked with severely ill AIDS patients for many years, and has increased T-cell counts from 210 to 270 with just three acupuncture treatments. 'One of these patients,' adds Dr Cargile, 'had a T-cell count of 30 to 40. We eventually brought it up to 270, and although that is half the level a person needs, he's been doing great for the last six months.'

Dr. Cargile adds that the key to understanding acupuncture's influence on blood values and cell counts lies in its ability to minimize stress and strengthen the body's adaptive mechanisms. 'I think that if we had more acupuncture and less drug medication, we would see a qualitative improvement in these patients' health.'

THREE WAYS OF HELPING?

Acupuncture is thought to assist the body in three different ways:

1 helping build the immune system back to strength
2 mobilizing the body's antiviral defenses
3 stimulating relaxation.

Chinese and Western research shows, for example, that a needle placed into a point below the knee (known as Tsu San Li or Stomach point 36) will increase white blood cell counts by up to 70 percent 3 hours later. And after a day the levels are still about 30 percent higher than before the acupuncture.

When non-acupuncture points are needled no rise in immune defense takes place – which demonstrates that the benefit observed is not a reaction to having needles placed just anywhere on the body surface.[87,88,89]

This is just one of literally hundreds of pieces of evidence supporting the immune-enhancing effects of acupuncture.

When 200 patients with immune depression were treated in New York, acupuncture was found to reduce levels of secondary opportunistic infections and to have a general beneficial influence.[90]

Drs. Smith and Rabinowitz, who conducted the research on patients at Lincoln Memorial Hospital, report that in some cases patients' T-cell ratios were seen to rise dramatically over a two- or three-month time scale using only acupuncture.

Acupuncture is a safe option to be seriously considered if you are in any way immune-compromised or even if you just want to maintain or improve an immune system which is working reasonably well.

7: Ecological Damage Caused by Antibiotics – The Yeast Connection[1,2,3,4,5]

We have seen in Chapter 4 that antibiotics, depending upon which class they are, produce a cluster of side-effects of varying intensity.

Many of these are avoidable if precautions are taken. Depending upon the particular drug, this might involve avoiding the use of particular types of antibiotics if kidney, liver or allergy problems have been noted in the past, or if the recipient is breastfeeding or pregnant.

Unlike these toxic side-effects, which are important to some patients but not others, and which relate to some antibiotics and not others, it is vital to realize that practically all antibiotics cause damage to some aspects of the normal flora of the body, simply because they are antibiotics.

The ecological havoc that results from such damage can seriously modify your internal ecology, with major health implications for years to come.

This is not just a matter of the development of oral or vaginal thrush after antibiotics – unpleasant as that may be – but of the chances of major damage occurring to the immune system, to the level of your health and quality of life.

This sort of damage could happen to you, so be aware of the dangers and do something about avoiding them, if you have to have antibiotics (*see Chapter 9*).

This sort of internal environmental change is not due to 'misuse' of antibiotics, but to their normal use, and although we have just looked at some strategies we might care to adopt in order to avoid the use of this class of drugs, there are most certainly times when antibiotics are essential.

At such times it is important to know how to reduce the internal ecological mayhem that is being wrought on your symbiotic, friendly bacteria (*see Chapter 2 for a reminder of the roles of the friendly bacteria*).

Let's consider the words and warnings of some leading authorities, both 'pro' and 'anti' antibiotics:

Dr. John Henry, Consultant Physician at Guy's Hospital and St. Thomas's Hospital, London, and chief medical editor for the *British Medical Association's New Guide to Medicines and Drugs* (London: Dorling Kindersley, 1995), who is anything but antagonistic to the use of antibiotics, says:

> *Another risk of antibiotic treatment, especially if it is prolonged, is that the balance of microorganisms normally inhabiting the body may be disturbed. In particular antibiotics may destroy bacteria that limit the growth of Candida, a yeast often present in the body in small amounts. This can lead to overgrowth of Candida (also known as thrush) in the mouth, vagina, or bowel.*

Note that Candida is not only 'often' present in the body, but is *always* present, and waiting for a chance to spread if this comes along, when and if normal controls (the friendly bacteria, for example) are weakened.

Professor Marc Lappe of the University of Illinois College of Medicine, in his book *When Antibiotics Fail* (Berkeley, CA: North Atlantic Press, 1995), who has campaigned against the overuse of antibiotics in food production and treatment of infection, says the following in relation to amoxycillin (although it applies to other antibiotics as well):

> *The most immediate impact of the very first doses of amoxycillin are felt in the intestine. There, many types of bacteria are drastically reduced in numbers. Some, like the*

Clostridium and Streptococcus varieties, rebound almost immediately – but with a difference. They are, at least for the short run, almost always resistant to the drug that is being used. More beneficial bacteria, like the milk-fermenting lactobacillus types, are almost always complete-ly destroyed. More resistant but less desirable bacteria includ-ing some with disease-causing abilities elsewhere in the body, begin to proliferate as more 'living room' is created by the death of their normal competitors. Among the new opportunists is a bad actor known as Candida albicans, a yeast that can cause serious infection of the vagina. Another is Clostridium difficile, a disease causing bacteria that can cause fatal inflammation of the lining of the intes-tine known as pseudomembranous colitis.

Lappe continues, later in the book,

Other antibiotics now alter intestinal flora with regularity. Lincomycin eliminates virtually all the bacteria that require oxygen, while neomycin and kanamycin decrease the num-ber of oxygen-requiring germs and the gram-positive anaerobic ones, leading to overgrowth of Candida albicans and Staphylococcus aureus … When cephalosporins are used in therapy there is a similarly dramatic shift in micro-flora particularly in the vagina.

Dr. Joseph Pizzorno, N.D., President of Bastyr University, Seattle, writing in his book *Total Wellness* (Rocklin, CA: Prima, 1996), reports on this phenomenon as follows:

In a study of 55 injured patients admitted to the trauma service of a hospital, all were given broad-spectrum anti-biotic therapy during some point of their stay. Sixty-seven per cent developed elevated Candida antigen levels in their blood during their hospital stay, indicating that Candida were overgrowing in their intestines (and the vagina in women). The researchers also found that the white blood cells of patients with Candida antigens were not able to inhibit Candida albicans growth as effectively as white blood cells from patients who did not have candidal antigens in their blood. In other words, when patients receive antibiotics, the level of Candida in their intestines increases so much, and the intestines become so damaged, that pieces of the Candida leak into their bloodstream and inhibit the function of their immune system.

Here we see that it is not just a matter of an additional yeast problem developing after antibiotic treatment – but an actual decrease in the efficiency of the immune defenses as well.

Awareness of this connection between antibiotic use and yeast overgrowth is not new. To show just how far back it was that doctors first understood and debated this connection, quotes are given below from a report by Doctors Huppert, MacPherson and Cazin, all from the Department of Bacteriology and Immunology, University of North Carolina School of Medicine, in 1952. They presented three theories as to why yeast overgrowth might take place after antibiotic treatment:

1/ Administration of antibiotics upsets the equilibrium in which the normal flora exists ... permitting the resistant species [yeasts, which of course are not susceptible to antibiotics] to increase vastly their population and thereby overwhelm the host resistance. 2/ The disturbance of the normal flora by antibiotic therapy, results in nutritional disturbance [most importantly deficiency of vitamin B, which the normal flora manufacture] which affects the integrity of the mucous membranes, opening a portal of entry for microorganisms which are normally unable to penetrate the intact healthy mucosa. 3/ Some of the antibiotics directly stimulate the growth and/or virulence of Candida albicans.

Natural Alternatives to Antibiotics

What is so fascinating about this report, which is almost half a century old, is that it was correct in all its thoughts as to what was happening – the normal bacteria which control yeast are damaged by antibiotics, and this allows yeast to overwhelm and colonize the bowel; because the normal flora can no longer manufacture B-vitamins (they also perform other functions such as maintaining the correct acidity levels) the bowel mucosa (lining) is damaged, allowing leakage into the blood of not just the yeasts but all sorts of toxic debris which can provoke allergic and toxic reactions; and there is evidence that Candida actually thrives on some antibiotics – such as Aureomycin.

Despite the knowledge of ecological damage highlighted by these extracts and quotes, very little is usually done by doctors to counter these negative antibiotic effects, despite methods being available to help reverse them. Hopefully a wider recognition of just how widespread the problems are that result from such damage will lead to action being taken and advice being given, along the lines set out in Chapters 9 and 10.

The Problems that Follow Yeast Overgrowth

Candida is known to be potentially very harmful because of its ability to turn from a simple yeast into an aggressive mycelial fungus which puts down 'rootlets' (rhizomes) into the mucous membrane of the intestinal tract, so permitting undesirable toxins to move from the bowel into the bloodstream, with the strong possibility of allergic and toxic reactions taking place as a result.

The many symptoms which have been catalogued in people affected in this way include:

○ a range of digestive symptoms (bloating, irritable bowel conditions involving swings from diarrhea to constipation and back to diarrhea)

- o chronic urinary tract infections
- o chronic and extreme unnatural fatigue
- o severe muscle aches (fibromyalgia)
- o emotional disturbances
- o 'foggy' brain symptoms
- o skin problems
- o menstrual problems
- o prostate problems
- o thrush (oral or vaginal)
- o fungal skin infections such as athlete's foot or ringworm, or fungal nail conditions.

The frequency with which such symptoms are suffered is enormous and may be related to a chronic yeast overgrowth – although other reasons are possible for almost all of them.

HOW CAN YOU TELL YEAST IS THE CAUSE?

Laboratory tests to 'prove' yeast involvement are commonly inaccurate, mainly because almost everyone on the planet has some yeast living in their digestive tract – simply finding it there does not help to determine just how widespread its presence is.

Diagnosis by symptoms (*see Questionnaire, below*) is more accurate: if an anti-Candida program (such as is described below) makes symptoms vanish or improve greatly, this confirms the diagnosis of yeast overgrowth.

One useful test, which requires a specialist laboratory, involves a sugar-loading test – a sample of blood is taken, then 100 grams of sugar are consumed on an empty stomach, then another blood sample is taken one hour later. This test assesses the levels of alcohol in the blood before and after the sugar intake, because yeast – and some bacteria – can turn sugar into alcohol rapidly in the intestines.

WHEN TO SUSPECT CANDIDA OVERGROWTH

Candida overgrowth may prove to be a factor in your health problems if after examining the lists below you find that one item or more from each applies to you.

(a) Have you:
- ○ a history of long-term antibiotic usage (one long period of taking them – more than two months – or more than four courses in any one year)? This would have damaged the normal flora and allowed the ever-present yeast to spread opportunistically.
- ○ ever taken a course of tetracycline (or any other antibiotic) to treat acne for more than one month?

(b) And, do you (or have you):
- ○ suffered from persistent prostatitis or cystitis or urethritis?
- ○ had ringworm or athlete's foot?
- ○ had cravings for sugar or bread or alcohol?

(c) And are you currently suffering from:
- ○ fatigue?
- ○ digestive bloating or 'irritable bowel'?
- ○ foggy brain (short-term memory difficulties, concentration problems)?
- ○ widespread muscular aches and pains?
- ○ thrush?
- ○ loss of sexual interest?

If you consider that you may have a Candida overgrowth, or if this has been diagnosed by a responsible health care professional, you may wish to consult an expert who deals with such problems, or to read more about it. (The book *Candida Albicans – Could Yeast Be Your Problem?* [Thorsons 1995] describes a comprehensive self-help program.)

Conditions associated with fungal infection, whether these involve the skin, the intestinal tract, or the urinary tract, may appear to be worse for the first few weeks of an anti-Candida diet.

Candidiasis and Immune Function

Recurrent candidiasis is common in people who are immune-compromised, and the condition can become almost universal and constant as immune efficiency declines.

Canadian naturopathic physician Eileen Stretch reports that unexplained vaginal candidiasis which is resistant to treatment is often the only clinical indication of severe underlying immunodeficiency.[6]

As yeast overgrowth progresses, in both men and women whose immune systems are compromised, the yeast often spreads to the mouth, larynx and pharynx, and sometimes to the stomach and esophagus.

One of the key results of chronic candidiasis is the damage caused to the intestinal walls, which allows absorption into the bloodstream of multiple antigenic and toxic substances, resulting in allergies which are commonly seen in people who have lowered immune function.

Dr. Eunice Carlson of Michigan University has shown that when Candida is actively present in the system at the same time as an infectious agent such as *Staphylococcus aureus*, the toxicity of the latter is enhanced by a huge amount and can result in fatal Toxic Shock Syndrome.[7]

DR. JESSOP'S EVIDENCE

San Francisco physician Carol Jessop has summarized the findings of her research into the backgrounds of over 1,300 of her patients suffering from chronic fatigue syndrome or fibromyalgia (FMS), a form of chronic muscle pain as well as fatigue.[8]

- ○ 82% of 880 patients tested had yeast cultured from purged stool samples.
- ○ 30% had parasites in their purged stool samples.
- ○ 38% were found to be deficient in magnesium.
- ○ 32% had low zinc levels.

Common symptoms found in Dr. Jessop's patients:

Chronic fatigue	100%
Cold extremities	100%
Impaired memory	100%
Frequent urination	95%
Depression	94%
Sleep disorders	94%
Balance problems	89%
Muscle twitching	80%
Dry mouth	68%
Muscle aches	68%
Headache	68%
Sore throat	20%

Dr. Jessop stated that patients were suffering a 'reactive depression' and not a 'clinical depression', and that only 8 percent of her depressed patients had required prior medical attention for this before the symptoms of CFS or FMS emerged. Quite simply, the patients were depressed because of their chronic pain and fatigue. These symptoms were not the result of depression but the cause of it.

Dr. Jessop reported that 87 percent of her 1,324 patients (average age 39, 75 percent female) had laboratory evidence of yeast infections (tongue/mouth).

Dr. Jessop's patients' symptoms *before* chronic fatigue (CFS) or muscle pain (FMS) symptoms had developed:

- ○ 89% had irritable bowel symptoms before their FMS/CFS.
- ○ 80% had 'constant gas' or bloating before their FMS/CFS.
- ○ 58% had constipation before their FMS/CFS.
- ○ 40% reported heartburn before their FMS/CFS.
- ○ 89% reported recurrent childhood ear, nose, throat infections.
- ○ 40% had a history of recurrent sinusitis.
- ○ 30% recurrent bronchitis before their FMS/CFS.
- ○ 20% recurrent bladder infections before their FMS/CFS.
- ○ 90% of the females had PMS symptoms before their FMS/CFS.
- ○ 65% reported endometriosis before their FMS/CFS.
- ○ 30% had dysmenorrhea before their FMS/CFS.
- ○ 22% had generalized anxiety disorders prior to their illness.
- ○ Sleep problems were present in only 1% before CFS/FMS.

She reports that 80 percent of the patients had a history of antibiotic treatment for ear, nose and throat infections, acne and/or urinary tract infections.

Sixty percent of her patients reported developing sensitivity to antibiotics.

A glance at the details of Dr. Jessop's summary of signs, symptoms and histories leads to a strong suggestion that antibiotics played a major part in the development of chronic yeast problems – which were themselves more than likely major players in the development of the symptom pictures which her patients displayed.

Medical treatment of the yeast may involve:

- ○ for local treatment – chlortrimazole
- ○ for bowel overgrowth – nystatin
- ○ for systemic involvement – fluconazole and itraconazole.

Most of these drugs have some side-effects, and highlight the chief flaw in the orthodox approach: while the antifungal drugs are being used, or immediately after this, little attention is paid to restoring the natural ecological balance in the body, which itself controls yeast.

This almost inevitably means that yeast overgrowth will return soon after antifungal drug treatment ceases, and the cycle will repeat itself.

ALTERNATIVE METHOD[9]

○ In order to avoid this repetitive cycle, unconventional medical approaches use a triple attack which attempts to kill the yeast using a variety of herbal products such as garlic, caprylic acid (coconut plant extract), aloe vera juice, Glycyrrhiza, hydrastis and/or echinacea.

○ At the same time, replenishment of bowel flora is attempted using proven viable colonizing strains of *L. acidophilus* and *Bifidobacteria*. These are the normal controlling element for Candida which are usually damaged when antibiotics or steroid drugs are used medically.[10] The dosages, etc. for such an approach are detailed in Chapter 9.

○ In addition, a general low-sugar/high-complex carbohydrate diet together with cultured (live) dairy products is suggested. Such methods are commonly extremely successful but may take six months or more to control the yeast overgrowth.

○ Alcohol also needs to be avoided as it is broken down (metabolized) in the body in much the same way as simple sugars and provides sustenance for yeast – encouraging it to grow.

○ The low-sugar diet is important because sugars encourage fermentation, which in turn encourages yeast activity. There are some sweet substances which do not have this effect, known as fructo-oligosaccharides (FOS), derived from Jerusalem artichokes and dandelion roots, which actually encourage the bifidobacteria without encouraging yeasts. FOS are available in powdered form from health food stores.

○ Some patients need also to abandon, for several months at least, all foods related to or containing yeasts or molds (including blue cheeses) because the body may have become sensitized to yeast or its byproducts.

THREE-MONTH BASIC ANTI-CANDIDA STRATEGY

Ideally to be undertaken only under supervision of an appropriately qualified and licensed health care professional.

1 Caprylic acid (antifungal coconut plant extract) – 1 capsule with each meal (that is, three times a day).
2 Biotin – 500 microgrammes (mcg) twice daily. This B vitamin helps to control the yeast's tendency to alter to a more aggressive form.
3 High-potency garlic – 1 capsule with each meal (three times a day). Antifungal, antibiotic.
4 Pau D'arco tea – three to four times daily.
5 Any of the following three herbs, individually or in combination:
  ○ *Hydrastis canandensis* (Goldenseal)
  ○ *Berberis vulgaris* (Barberry) and/or
  ○ *Echinacea angustifolia* (Purple Coneflower)
  ○ – three times daily as an antifungal, antibacterial, immune-enhancing support.
  ○ These herbs should be obtained from a reputable herbal supplier or health food store and used according to the instructions on the pack. For more details regarding them individually, see Chapter 6.

Note
Many other antifungal substances are available and may be more effective in certain cases than the suggestions above, which are however usually beneficial if the program is maintained for several months.

Encouraging Repopulation of Intestinal Flora

O High-quality *acidophilus* and *Bifidobacteria* (powder or capsule form) – between meals (three times daily), either a capsule of each or between one-quarter and a whole teaspoon of powdered versions of each, as well as *L. bulgaricus* – as discussed in Chapter 9.

O General nutritional support is useful – taking a well-formulated, yeast-free, hypoallergenic multi-vitamin/ multimineral to provide at least the recommended daily allowance of major nutrients.

DIETARY SUGGESTIONS FOR CANDIDA

O Chew well/eat slowly/try not to drink much with meals.

O Eat three small main meals daily as well as two snack meals where possible (no sugar-rich food), or take 3 to 5 grams of full-spectrum amino acid complex between main meals, twice daily.

O Include in the diet as much ginger, cinnamon, and garlic (as well as other aromatic herbs, such as oregano) as possible – all are antifungal and most also aid digestive processes.

O To assist with bowel function, regularly (daily, same time every day) take at least 1 tablespoonful of linseed. Swallow with water, unchewed, to provide a soft fiber to assist intestinal emptying.

O Avoid as far as possible all refined sugars and for the first few weeks avoid very sweet fruit as well (melon, sweet grapes). Avoid aged cheeses, dried fruits and any food obviously derived from or containing yeast (in case of sensitization).

O Avoid caffeine (coffee, tea, chocolate, cola, etc.) as this produces a sugar release which is not desirable where yeast has proliferated.

O Avoid alcohol.

○ If possible avoid all yeast-based foods – including bread and anything that has included yeast in its manufacture or which might contain mold.

You may feel off-color for the first week of such a program as yeast 'die-off' (Herxheimer's reaction) takes place. This will pass on its own, however anyone with a severe and longstanding yeast problem might consider supplementing with high doses of probiotics for a week or so before starting the anti-Candida program to reduce the intensity of the 'die-off' reaction.

Summary

○ Antibiotics, to a greater or lesser extent, damage the internal flora of the intestinal tract, upon which our health (and lives) depend.
○ Opportunistic yeasts (and other undesirable microbes) colonize areas vacated by weakened or dead friendly bacteria, which normally control them.
○ Yeasts (and other undesirable microbes) can produce major changes to the health of the lining of the intestines, damaging it and allowing passage into the bloodstream of undesirable toxins and proteins.
○ A wide range of symptoms can then emerge as the immune system tries to cope with this onslaught.
○ There exist safe, effective, and proven strategies for reducing the likelihood of this happening, and of reversing the damage if it does happen.
○ The opportunity to prevent or reverse this risk (of yeast overgrowth) exists for adults and children (*see Chapters 9 and 10*).

8: Antibiotics, Bowel Flora, and Illness

A survey of the conditions in the previous chapter which summarized Dr. Jessop's findings (repeated below) gives a strong clue as to the sort of ailments which might feature antibiotics as one of the culprits. This survey of over 1,300 of her patients showed that over 80 percent had a history of lengthy or repetitive antibiotic use, with 60 percent developing allergy to antibiotics. Most had severe or complicated bowel problems – almost always involving yeast overgrowth (superinfection) plus a host of associated conditions – including fatigue, muscle pain, and allergic tendencies. Their most prominent symptoms were:

Chronic fatigue	100%
Cold extremities	100%
Impaired memory	100%
Frequent urination	95%
Depression	94%
Sleep disorders	94%
Balance problems	89%
Muscle twitching	80%
Dry mouth	68%
Muscle aches	68%
Headache	68%
Sore throat	20%

Additionally, Dr. Jessop recorded the following major problems prior to the patients' consulting her for their chronic fatigue and muscle pain (fibromyalgia) symptoms:

Premenstrual syndrome	90%
Irritable bowel	89%
Recurrent history of ear, nose and throat infections	89%
Bloating and gas	80%
Endometriosis	65%
Constipation	58%
Heartburn	40%
Recurrent sinusitis	40%
Recurrent bronchitis	30%
Dysmenorrhea	30%
Recurrent bladder infections	20%

We can see from the histories of these patients that the digestive tract was very much involved; as we have seen in previous chapters, this region is an obvious and vulnerable target for the damage caused by many of the different forms of antibiotic.

Once the friendly flora populations of the digestive tract are damaged – by toxicity, a high-fat/high-sugar diet, and/or by antibiotics – a range of conditions can arise relating to the functions they perform, including increased toxicity for the liver to try and deal with.

The conditions discussed below are illustrative of some of the serious and not so serious health repercussions associated with antibiotics. This brief survey is not fully comprehensive, since it is meant to highlight the interplay between normal function, often involving the friendly bacteria, and the effects of antibiotics.

Liver Disease

Because the friendly bacteria detoxify the bowel and help the liver in its detoxification tasks, once the bowel flora has been compromised the liver may become overloaded (*see Chapter 7*). We have already seen (*Chapter 4*) just how many of the antibiotics can be involved in liver disease, and the precautions which are called for. It is absolutely certain that in many cases a major part of this increased risk and damage to the liver is the result of the weakened role of the normal flora, and the increased toxic load the liver has to cope with.

Restoring the flora (*see Chapters 9 and 10 for guidelines*) will undoubtedly help liver function, no matter how serious the problem.

Evidence for this statement can be found in a number of studies and reports involving people (some of them children) with severe cirrhosis of the liver or hepatitis (liver inflammation) where it was found that supplementation with bifidobacteria (sometimes for only 7 to 10 days) as well as a bifidogenic diet (a diet, as described in Chapter 7, page 165, which supports the friendly bacteria) dramatically lowered the levels of toxic ammonia and other toxins (phenols, etc.) in the bloodstream to almost normal levels and assisted in the recovery or stabilization of many of the patients.[1,2]

Acne

This common skin condition attracts a high degree of antibiotic use which can produce severe and long-term repercussions. As Dr. Jessop noted in her research, antibiotic use was a common predisposing feature of most of her patients.

Professor Marc Lappe reports that *Propionibacterium acnes*, a bacterium which lives harmlessly on our skin in huge numbers, has been blamed (mistakenly, he believes) for acne.[3]

He says,

> This bacterium is particularly hard hit by tetracycline, a drug championed by those who see acne as a problem calling for an antibiotic solution. Unfortunately, as these benign compatriots wane, their place is rapidly filled by staph microbes that quickly develop resistance to the

tetracycline. Still other bacteria, notably Micrococcus luteus which holds the first line of defence in the skin against Staphylococcus aureus, die off and leave the field open for a potential overgrowth of antibiotic resistant staph.

Lappe, who is no fringe cult quack but a highly respected professor of medicine at the University of Illinois' College of Medicine, argues that this approach is 'mediaeval and messy' (and he is quoting from a 1979 issue of a major British medical journal, the *Lancet*).

He goes on to describe a 1980 issue of the *Journal of the American Medical Association* which reported on the testing of three different approaches to acne treatment:

1 16 weeks on tetracycline antibiotics combined with cleansing agents for the skin
2 16 weeks of tetracycline plus another drug, tretinoin, which reduced fatty acids in the skin
3 16 weeks using tretinoin to reduce fatty acids along with a soothing unguent (benzoyl peroxide).

The results showed that the non-antibiotic approach (option 3) was as good or better than either of the antibiotic approaches in terms of improvement of acne – and without the devastation which tetracycline can cause to the internal ecology of the body.

There are, of course, other ways of handling acne without using drugs at all: nutritional strategies are high on the list of helpful methods.

Dietary Strategies

○ First it is necessary to reduce carbohydrate intake, especially of sugars, and to increase protein intake to adequate levels, not less than 3 oz (90 g) daily.
○ In normalizing severe acne, the health of the bowels is vital. Research in Baltimore showed that supplementing

with acidophilus alone could benefit acne patients. In treating over 300 cases, *L. acidophilus* and *L. bulgaricus* (*see Chapter 9*) were supplemented three times daily. The period of time involved ranged from 2 weeks to 3 months, after which 80 percent of the patients reported success, half of these saying the changes were 'excellent' and the other half that the improvements were 'reasonable.'

○ No other changes were made aside from the probiotic supplementation, and it is suggested that this approach, together with the dietary methods listed below, would produce far better results.

○ People with acne should avoid foods containing iodine (such as seaweed, which also means kelp tablets), as research shows that this substance aggravates the condition.

○ Animal fats should be severely restricted because of the harm they do generally as well as the problems they cause in the digestive tract – and the damage they do to the friendly bacteria.

○ In order to help the body deal better with carbohydrates, a chromium supplement is often needed (400 micrograms daily is suggested). This helps to keep blood sugar levels stable, something very important in any effort to keep undesirable bacteria and yeasts from proliferating.

○ Vitamin A in high doses is helpful, but high-dosage supplementation should not be undertaken without supervision and so is not recommended as part of any self-help program. It is safe to take up to 20,000 iu daily without supervision.

○ Zinc is also useful in acne, as in so many other skin problems. It is involved in local hormone activation as well as control of vitamin A activity, wound healing, and tissue regeneration (20 to 40 mg daily is suggested).

○ Together with zinc, vitamin B_6 is needed, as these work together in many of the bodily processes. This is especially true if acne is worse before or during menstrual periods. 100 mg daily is suggested.

○ Vitamin E and selenium have an influence on acne and are suggested as regular supplements to the diet (400 iu of E and 200 micrograms of selenium are recommended).

○ Dietary changes might also include the use of acidophilus and the supplemental nutrients as discussed in the anti-Candida diet in Chapter 7.

ACNE AND STRESS REDUCTION

In trials on severely affected teenagers in Florida, it was found that regular relaxation exercises reduced the incidence of acne dramatically. Over a three-month period those youngsters using simple relaxation techniques had better overall results than those who had regular medical care. Over a one-year follow-up, those who kept the exercises going (15 to 20 minutes a day) maintained their improvement, whereas those who stopped had relapses. Interestingly it has been shown that when we are highly stressed the changes which occur in digestive circulation as well as digestive enzyme and acid production have a seriously damaging effect on the normal flora of the intestines.

High Cholesterol Levels

The friendly bacteria which inhabit our intestines play a major part in processing bile and cholesterol in the bowels.

When they are healthy they perform these tasks as part of their normal activities. If they are not working well, and this can be because of excessive antibiotic use or because of a high-sugar, high-fat diet which doesn't suit them any more than it suits us, they cannot perform their recycling and detoxification duties efficiently. Yogurt is a natural food for the lactobacilli and the bifidus bacteria, and the benefits which have been reported regarding the lowering of high cholesterol levels when yogurt is regularly consumed (especially if it is low-fat and 'live') may relate to improvements which yogurt encourages in friendly bacteria activity.[4]

While excessive levels of some forms of cholesterol are obviously dangerous to the body, we cannot live without this wax-like material, which is part of every cell in the body. The friendly bacteria living in our intestines have a remarkable ability to break down and alter a number of essential substances which find their way into the bowel, including hormones such as estrogen (discussed later in this chapter) and the vital substance cholesterol.

A research study in 1979 first showed this remarkable function of the friendly bacteria. Fifty-four volunteers (24 men and 30 women), all in good health and with no history of either heart or gall bladder disease, were evaluated for 12 weeks. During this time they consumed specific amounts of either milk or yogurt. At the same time, another group of volunteers also had their diet supplemented with milk or yogurt, as well as live cultures of lactobacillus bulgaricus and thermophilus (the yogurt cultures – *described further in Chapter 9*).

Probably the most important finding from this study was that a significant reduction in cholesterol levels was noted in people receiving the live yogurt and live bacterial cultures – and that this benefit was noted after just 7 days.

Not only was there a reduction to healthier levels of blood cholesterol in these people, but the amount of 'new' cholesterol being made was reduced because 'old' cholesterol reaching the intestines in the bile was able to be recycled. Anyone with liver or gall bladder problems, or high cholesterol levels – or who simply wish their cholesterol levels to remain at healthy levels – should consider the regular use of live low-fat yogurt in their diet, as well as supplementation of friendly bacteria – as outlined in Chapter 9.[5,6]

The implications regarding cholesterol levels, if the friendly flora are damaged by antibiotics or anything else, are obvious. The recycling process described above is only effective if the flora are healthy; this cannot be the case if antibiotics are used either excessively or inappropriately.

Menopausal and Menstrual Problems

A glance back at the symptoms displayed by Dr. Jessop's unhappy collection of patients (*Chapter 7 and above*) shows us that most had a history of antibiotic overuse, the majority were women, and of these the bulk demonstrated evidence of yeast overgrowth accompanied by menstrual or menopausal irregularities.

As we have seen, when operating normally and not under assault by antibiotics, the friendly bacteria play a major part in maintaining normal cholesterol levels.

In much the same way the friendly bacteria 'filter' female (and, research now indicates, male) hormones which find themselves in the bowel, and return them to the bloodstream.

In this way the bowel flora have a major effect on estrogen, progesterone and androgen hormone levels. Researchers in the U.S. have shown just how powerful this influence can be.

Drs. Gary Simons and Sherwood Gorbach report, 'Several studies have demonstrated that approximately 60 percent of circulating estrogens [female sex hormones] are excreted in the bile.' Their report goes on to tell us that the estrogens are then 'processed' by the intestinal microflora (if they are functioning normally) so that in a healthy individual fully 97 percent of this estrogen is reclaimed ('deconjugated') and recycled back into the body.[7]

The effect of antibiotics on this important function is well established, showing that a significant degree of loss of estrogen occurs after antibiotic use. The researchers inform us that when antibiotics (including ampicillin, penicillin, chloramphenicol, sulfamethoxypyridazine and neomycin) are administered this process of reclaiming estrogen is severely disrupted, leading to up to 60 times more estrogen actually being eliminated in the urine or via bowel movements than would normally occur.

These researchers also inform us that antibiotics produce 'similar but not identical' effects on the way the body recycles progesterone, another female sex hormone, and that when antibiotics such as ampicillin are given to men, the amounts of certain male hormones are found to be dramatically increased in the feces.

What implications can this have on the health of the women (and in the case of androgens, the men) affected?

The research reports that there are several major implications which have been identified:

○ Because of the disruption of hormone balance, break-through bleeding may occur.
○ Pregnancy may occur due to antibiotic interference, via the friendly bacteria, with the hormones contained in con-traceptive pills.
○ We can add to these two possibilities a wide range of hor-mone-related disturbances which could emerge from such imbalances, including osteoporosis and a variety of men-strual and menopausal symptoms.
○ Quite simply, antibiotics can damage the bowel flora, so pre-venting hormone recycling and resulting in excessive loss of calcium, increased fragility of the bones and the danger of easy fracture, as well as creating imbalances which cause or aggravate menstrual and gynecological problems.[7,8]

All of these problems can be helped by normalizing the bowel flora, as outlined in Chapter 9.

Ankylosing Spondylitis,[8] Rheumatoid Arthritis, and Other Auto-immune Conditions

These conditions all seem to involve a case of 'mistaken identity.' They are all what are called auto-immune conditions, in which the immune system, for no obviously apparent reason, starts to attack parts of itself.

Diligent research has shown that when the normal flora of the intestines are damaged, involving particular bacteria in the overgrowth which then occurs (*see Chapter 7 for details of yeast overgrowth*) and – most importantly – when the protein 'tissue type' of the particular bacteria is very similar to that of the person him- or herself, the immune system mistakes its own tissues for those of the foreign bacteria and attacks itself.

When ankylosing spondylitis (AS) develops, a slow fusing occurs of the spine and pelvic joints, leading to what is called 'bamboo spine' and leaving the person affected stooped and stiff.

The bacteria thought to be involved in this is Klebsiella, commonly found in small numbers in the bowels of most people, but in superabundance in most people with AS. The tissue type designated as B27 is found in fully 98 percent of people with AS – and is the protein tissue type of Klebsiella as well.

Dr. Alan Ebringer of Kings College Hospital in London, having made the connection between Klebsiella and AS, decided to investigate a dietary approach to its control.

He explains,

> *Klebsiella thrives on a diet rich in starch [carbohydrates]. If you cut out starchy carbohydrates such as rice, potatoes and flour products, then you reduce the number of klebsiella in the gut, and subsequently the production of antibodies to the bacteria which cause the inflammation.*

Patients are given instructions to cut out bread, pasta, cereals of all sorts, rice and potatoes, as well as sugary foods. They can eat as much fruit, vegetables, eggs, cheese, fish, and meat as they like.

DOES THE DIET WORK?

The first 200 patients who completed the trial have had their disease process halted – normally this condition is progressive.

A similar connection has now been made in patients with that most destructive and crippling of destructive joint conditions, rheumatoid arthritis (RA).

Most people who develop RA possess the tissue type HLA-DR4, as does the bacterial organism Proteus, which is found in abundance in the intestines of most patients with RA. Significantly there is in many of these patients a history of bladder infections caused by Proteus and previously treated with antibiotics.

Unlike the sensible AS dietary strategy, researchers have suggested powerful antibiotic treatment to destroy these bacteria – an approach which seems odd, considering the way the condition developed in the first place.

Here once again we can see how bowel ecology can be modified – possibly by antibiotic use – leading to bacterial overgrowth and, in these particular conditions, the provocation of auto-immune attacks on the body.

And once again, in the example of Ankylosing spondylitis, we can see how a simple dietary approach can control the process.[9]

Dietary Treatment of E. coli Bladder Infections in Women[10]

In this instance we are not looking at a condition caused by antibiotics but at one in which their use may not be successful, or may become repetitive, with all the negative impact this can have, as noted by Dr. Jessop's research.

We will also examine a possible dietary solution developed in 1976 by doctors at Sefton Hospital, Liverpool, England. They suggested a diet (similar to that detailed in Chapter 7) to treat women who had repeated episodes of cystitis involving a bacteria normally found in the bowel, E. coli.

They report,

It is well established that urinary-tract infections are caused by the bowel type of organism and when the urinary tract is colonised, the faecal reservoir (the bacteria in the bowel) is the source of the infection, for example in hospital patients the strain of E. coli cultured in the urine can also be found in the faeces.

The women in the study had symptoms of either frequency of urination, or incontinence – being unable to control their bladder function at times. Antibiotics were used repeatedly and without benefit, no doubt causing an enormous degree of increased yeast activity which would almost certainly have made the bladder problems worse.

As the researchers put it,

Antibiotics may not relieve the symptoms, or recurrence occurs once the treatment is stopped, and complications may arise with bacterial resistance and toxic effects or monilial [yeast] infection following antibiotics.

They report that the distress of this condition is great and that a dietary strategy was commonly successful. The method, they claim, aims to reduce refined carbohydrates (sugars, alcohol, white bread, etc.) in order to 'starve' the disease-causing bacteria. The protocol recommended involves:

○ reduction of refined carbohydrates (a sugar-free, high-fiber diet)
○ the application of (iodine-based) disinfectant on the affected area
○ in stubborn cases – especially following use of antibiotics where yeast overgrowth is suspected – they report that the taking of Lactobacillus and/or yogurt is helpful
○ regular use of a bidet or hand-held shower to wash the region is encouraged (the towel used to wipe the area should be boiled regularly).

This is a very simple regime, offering extremely good results, and it has clear dietary similarities to the more complicated Candida regime described in Chapter 5. The doctors report that,

> When the regimen was introduced it was regarded with some scepticism by many nurses and doctors' wives who suffered recurrent frequency and dysuria. Nevertheless these patients have now become enthusiastic propagandists for the methods.

Complementary methods for treating chronic cystitis include:

○ The use of Cranberry juice, which reduces the ability of bacteria to adhere to the bladder wall (or that of the urethra). When consumed along with a high water intake the bacteria are literally flushed out of the system. Most commercial cranberry juice has a high sugar content; only sugar-free versions are suggested. A safer method is to take freeze-dried cranberry juice, which all health stores will supply either in capsule or powdered form. A teaspoon of this (or several capsules) taken twice daily should rapidly assist in eliminating all but the most stubborn bladder infections.

○ Supplementation with very high doses of vitamin C – however, since the type of vitamin C suggested will vary with the relative state of acidity of the urine, the details of this approach cannot be given here. Anyone who is interested in such an approach should consult a qualified naturopathic practitioner or someone well versed in nutritional medicine.

○ A research study involving 153 elderly women over a 6-month period indicated that 'use of cranberry beverage (300 ml daily) reduces frequency of bacteriuria and pyuria in older women'.[11] Blueberry extracts have a similar effect.[12]

Whether we are evaluating acne, osteoporosis or ankylosing spondylitis, or considering cystitis or cholesterol levels – there is in the background a connection between the health of the bowel flora and antibiotic overuse.

This connection is not to be found in every case, of course, but in a significant number a link is both possible and provable.

Should we therefore stop using antibiotics? No, of course not, but we should start using them sparingly, precisely and with the knowledge that they cause damage as well as saving lives, even when used correctly.

We can do a lot to reduce this damage, and the chain reaction of problems which can follow, by

O carefully paying attention to the marvelous bowel flora
O carrying out reflorastation of the bowel when the friendly bacteria are damaged
O employing safe techniques, perhaps involving diet, herbs, or other methods (*see Chapters 5 and 6*) in order to enhance immune function and discourage bacterial and other pathogenic organisms, without creating further problems for the body.

Gastric and Duodenal Ulcers

In 1983 it was found that over 70 percent of gastric ulcers were caused by a bacteria, *helicobacter pylori*. This bacteria burrows into the lining of the stomach or duodenum and creates irritation that leads to gastritis and, eventually, to ulcers. Standard medical treatment is to use a combination of antibiotics (chosen from metronidazole, tetracycline, amoxycillin, clarithromycin and azithromycin) along with powerful antacid. This is usually successful but leads to all the usual negative effects of antibiotic treatment. In many patients *H. pylori* is now found to have become resistant to antibiotics. Even more worrying is the fact that the World Health Organization now considers *H. pylori* to be one of the major causes of stomach cancer.

Alternative approaches have been tried using cranberries, garlic, cinnamon, thyme and liquorice, which can all suppress *H. pylori* to some extent. However the most successful alternative has been found in an ancient Greek remedy, natural chewing gum – mastic. Mastic gum is the sap taken from a small evergreen tree, *Pistacia lentiscus*, which grows wild in the Mediterranean region, mainly on the Greek island of Chios. Mastic has been used since classical times as an indigestion cure and is mentioned in hundreds of ancient medical books. Recent research studies[13,14] have shown that between 1 and 2 grams of mastic, taken daily as a supplement for just a few weeks, heals ulcers and completely deactivates *H. pylori* in almost three-quarters of people with ulcers – even when the bacteria had been shown to be resistant to antibiotics.

Other studies suggest that mastic gum can also inhibit the growth of other bacteria, such as *Staphylococcus aureus* and *Escherichia coli* as well as the bacteria responsible for dental plaque. In the UK mastic gum powder is available in supplement form (marketed as Mastika).

9: Probiotics – What to Do If You Have to Take Antibiotics

The friendly bacteria are also known as 'probiotics', which literally means 'for life', compared with antibiotics whose name means 'against life.'

It should by now have become clear that among the many things that can happen with antibiotic use is the likelihood of damage to the friendly bacteria living inside our digestive tract. The dangers this can represent to your health are enormous.

The most important strategies you can adopt if you are obliged to have a course of antibiotics are to ensure that you finish the course, and actively and sufficiently to replenish your friendly bacteria (known as the 'flora' of the gut).

You cannot live without these friendly bacteria (please refer again to the summary of their activities in Chapters 2 and 7), and when they are working at less than their efficient best (as they would be after a course of antibiotics) all sorts of associated health problems can arise.[1]

We have previously met the main cast of friendly bacteria and have noted their benefits, what can harm them, and the ways in which such changes can impact on health. In this chapter we will discover what we can do to maintain (or restore) the good health of these friendly bacteria, so that they can continue to perform the vital roles they play in our lives. The main focus of this chapter, therefore, is to learn how to help these life-saving probiotic organisms which live in us, work for us, and whose lives are so intimately bound up with our own.

Natural Alternatives to Antibiotics

The Friendly Bacteria[2]

Before we examine the benefits these bacteria offer and the health problems which can develop if they are damaged, we should once again, briefly, meet them individually (their primary functions are described in Chapter 2).

Bifidobacterium bifidum	inhabiting the intestines – with a greater presence in the large intestine (the colon) than in the small intestine. They also live in the vagina.
Lactobacillus acidophilus	main site of occupation is the small intestine. Also lives in the mouth and vagina.
Bifidobacterium longum	a natural inhabitant of the human intestines and vagina. Found in larger numbers in the large intestine than the small intestine. Together with other bifidobacteria, this is the dominant organism of breastfed infants (making up 99 percent of the microflora). In adolescence and adult life the bifidobacteria remain (when health is good) the dominant organism of the large intestine.
Bifidobacterium infantis	a natural inhabitant of the human infant's digestive tract (as well as of the vagina, in small quantities). Its presence is far greater in the bowel of breastfed infants compared with bottle-fed infants.
Lactobacillus bulgaricus	not a resident of the human body, but a 'transient.' Once it enters the body through food (yogurt, for example) it remains for several weeks before being passed, but while it is in the body it

	performs useful tasks, including 'helping' our main resident bacteria – acidophilus and bifidobacteria – to attach themselves to the lining of the intestines so that they can start to perform their vital cleansing and protective roles.
Streptococcus thermophilus	This is a transient (non-resident) bacteria of the human intestine which together with L. bulgaricus (*see above*) is a yogurt culture, also found in some cheeses.
Streptococcus faecium	a natural resident of the human intestine. It is found in human feces as well as on some plants and insects.

Some additional (useful) lactobacilli found in the digestive tract include:

the transient bacteria of the intestines: *L. casei, L. plantarum, L. brevis, L. delbrueckii,* and *L. caucasicus* (known as *L. kefir*) *L. salivarius* – a natural resident of the mouth and digestive tract.

Streptococcus faecalis	This is a resident of the human intestine which is known as an enterococcus. It is found in feces, some insects and some plants. It can produce toxic materials and has the potential to become a hostile bacteria.

Here is a summary of the benefits offered by the friendly bacteria – *when they are healthy*:[3,4,5]

O Improve the body's ability to digest milk products by producing the enzyme lactase

○ Aid digestive function overall and improve the body's ability to digest and absorb nutrients from food
○ Improve bowel function – when they are not healthy, bowel transit time (how long it takes food to be processed and wastes to be eliminated) is far slower
○ Some strains can destroy invading bacteria by producing natural antibiotic products
○ Some strains have anti-tumor effects
○ By acting to detoxify the intestines (preventing amine formation, for example) they help to prevent the formation of cancer-causing chemicals
○ Decrease the levels of cholesterol in the system, so reducing the dangers which excess cholesterol poses to the health of the heart and circulatory system
○ Some strains assist in recycling estrogen, which helps overall hormone balance as well as reducing menopausal symptoms
○ Manufacture some of the B-vitamins including B_3, B_6, folic acid, and biotin
○ Maintain control over potentially hostile yeasts such as Candida albicans
○ Produce lactic acid, which enhances the digestibility of foods as well as improving the environment for friendly bacteria and making it hostile for invading organisms. For example, they protect against most of the organisms which produce food poisoning.

WHAT DISTURBS THE FRIENDLY BACTERIA?[6,7,8,9,10]

(See Chapter 10 for discussion of how this applies to infants and children.)

The natural balance and population levels of friendly bacteria in the body can be upset by:

- many drugs, the most obvious being antibiotics, steroids (cortisone and prednisone, for example) and chemotherapy drugs
- anything at all which causes a gastric (stomach) upset, whether this is stress, smoking, undesirable food combinations, or anything else
- anything which alters the normal function of the bowel – either slowing it down (constipation) or speeding it up (colitis, diarrhea, etc.)
- anything which reduces the levels of normal digestive acids in the stomach, which decline with age anyway (as they also do if we are zinc-deficient)
- pernicious anemia (which is associated with lowered stomach acid levels)
- a toxic state of the bowel – as occurs with chronic constipation, for example
- a high-fat diet
- a high-sugar diet
- smoking
- excess alcohol
- emotional stress
- environmental pollutants (pesticides, petrochemicals, heavy metals such as lead, mercury, cadmium, etc.)
- damage to the internal lining of the intestines, such as occurs in colitis, regional enteritis, diverticulitis and Crohn's disease
- exposure to radiation (including x-rays)
- liver disease, such as cirrhosis
- immune deficiency – produced by infection (e.g. HIV) or drugs (e.g. as used in transplant surgery to reduce the chances of organ rejection)
- most chronic disease.

Famed medical researcher René Dubos maintains that the most important elements which upset the friendly bacteria are the foods we eat, our stress levels, and the drugs (antibiotics, etc.) we use.[11]

DISEASES ASSOCIATED WITH DAMAGED BOWEL FLORA

Note

This is only a partial list, since almost all conditions of the human body may feature some aspect of bowel dysfunction as an associated factor.

○ Acne, which is commonly associated with a bowel dysbiosis – an unhealthy, toxic state of the intestines which probiotic use can help to reduce.

○ All allergic conditions which are associated with foods may have as a cause reduced bowel flora efficiency, for several reasons. If the bowel mucosa are irritated the bowel can become 'leaky' and allow passage through it, to the bloodstream, of substances which will provoke an allergic reaction. The 'leaky bowel' can be helped by probiotic supplementation – as well as other nutritional, medical and herbal strategies. Allergy can also be aggravated by the production of excessive amounts of histamine, which some bacteria can produce when the flora is unbalanced.

○ Auto-immune diseases such as rheumatoid arthritis, Lupus, and Ankylosing spondylitis in which particular associated bacteria are excessively present (for example Proteus in the case of rheumatoid arthritis, Klebsiella in Ankylosing spondylitis). *(See Chapter 8 for more on these conditions.)* All these bacteria can be controlled by the normal flora when it is in good health.

○ Bladder infections become more likely when the normal bowel flora are damaged or operating inefficiently for any of the reasons listed above.

○ High cholesterol levels. We make most of our own cholesterol, with only about 15 percent coming from the diet. Cholesterol is not just one substance but comes in 'good' and 'bad' (and 'very bad') forms. The friendly bacteria act to salvage and recycle good (high-density) cholesterol which would otherwise be excreted through the bowels.

○ The heart and cardiovascular system are therefore protected if the friendly bacteria are in good health (*also see Chapter 8*).

○ Irritable bowel problems (IBS) are commonly associated with bowel flora damage which has led to yeast or bacterial overgrowth in territories usually occupied by the friendly bacteria.

○ The detoxifying powers of healthy bowel flora reduce the chances of cancer-forming substances being created in the intestines. If these chemicals (nitrites, etc.) are allowed to form because of bowel flora inefficiency, cancer could be provoked.

○ Candida albicans overgrowth, which can produce IBS, also produces oral and vaginal thrush. It has been shown that treating the local outbreak of yeast infection (in the mouth, for example) without also dealing with what is happening in the bowel will not control the situation for more than a short time (*also see Chapter 7*). Candida is also linked to the development of the 'leaky bowel' syndrome mentioned above.

○ Colitis, a chronic inflammation of the lower bowel, can often be helped by supplementation with friendly bacteria.

○ Chronic fatigue syndrome (CFS, also known in the UK as ME) has been shown to be directly associated, in many cases, with a history of bowel dysbiosis and/or candidiasis – both of which are linked to a weakened state of the normal bowel flora.

○ Food poisoning becomes more likely when the normal flora is damaged, since the majority of food poisoning organisms can be easily controlled by *L. acidophilus* and/or the bifidobacteria when they are operating normally.

○ Liver diseases can be helped by friendly bacteria which reduce the toxic load that this vital organ has to handle.

○ Menopausal problems. Not just hot flashes but potentially dangerous problems such as osteoporosis are minimized by the salvaging and recycling of estrogen (which would otherwise be excreted) by the friendly bacteria (*also see Chapter 8*).

○ Migraine headaches can be triggered by excessive amounts of the chemical tyramine, which some bacteria can produce when the flora is unbalanced.

○ Chronic muscular pain, such as fibromyalgia, has been shown to be directly associated, in most cases, with a history of bowel dysbiosis and/or candidiasis – both of which are linked to a weakened state of the normal bowel flora.

Many of the conditions listed above also involve extreme distress, anxiety and depression, and have a terrible impact on a person's life and ability to function normally.

Probiotic Nutritional Guidelines

So what do the friendly bacteria like, and what don't they like?

Foods and substances which improve the health of the friendly bacteria, or which encourage their ability to colonize (attach to the lining of the bowel) and thrive, so that they can provide the many benefits they offer us in return for accommodation – are called bifidogenic foods.

○ Complex carbohydrates – such as fresh vegetables, pulses (the bean family, including lentils, soya beans, etc.), nuts, seeds, whole grains (wheat, rice, oats, etc.) are all bifidogenic – they are welcomed by the friendly bacteria because they offer just the sort of nourishment needed.

○ Particular vegetables which have been shown to help bifidobacteria function include carrots, potatoes, and maize extracts.

○ Fermented milk products – kefir, sour milk, cottage cheese, yogurt, etc. – are the perfect bifidogenic food for the lactobacilli and the bifidobacteria, but these must not contain antibiotic residues which are present in many commercial dairy foods. This calls for extra expense and effort, if possible, in tracking down sources which guarantee that the herds from which the dairy products come are 'organic' or 'free range' or 'chemical free.' Goat and sheep's milk products are usually (but not always) chemical free. Fermented soya products – tofu and miso, for example – are almost as good as dairy foods.

○ Low-fat meats and fish are good foods for the friendly bacteria. Meat and fish which are 'factory farmed' are likely to have antibiotic residues – so look for organic or free-range poultry and meat, and non-farmed fish.

○ Removing the fat from milk and replacing it with a vegetable source of oil, such as is found in flax seed oil, enhances bifidobacteria function.

○ Lactulose – a combination of fruit sugar and galactose created by heating milk – is also bifidogenic. Lactulose is used by doctors when liver function is poor, to help bifidobacteria to reduce the load on the liver.

When it comes to what the friendly bacteria don't like, refined carbohydrates (sugars, white flour products) and high-fat foods are top of the list. In addition, they respond badly to sustained stress, as this produces biochemical changes in the intestines, in terms of hormonal changes and alterations in the production of digestive acids and enzymes.

In summary, then, the best way forward is to reduce stress levels and eat a diet which emphasizes low-fat, low-sugar, high-complex carbohydrate, useful levels of cultured and fermented dairy (and other products) such as yogurt and tofu, and to avoid toxic and antibiotic residues in food.

To give a real boost to friendly bacteria function, consider supplementing with the main probiotic organisms: *L. acidophilus*, the bifidobacteria, and *L. bulgaricus*.

PROBIOTIC REPLENISHMENT

Whenever purchasing a probiotic product, try to ensure the following (*see separate guidelines for purchasing probiotics for infants in Chapter 10*):

○ The product should ideally contain only one organism – a single type of friendly bacteria – not a cocktail. However, if more than one organism is present in a capsule or container, ensure that the label contains a statement telling you the minimum numbers of each organism, not just their names.

○ Ensure that the names of the organisms in the container are clearly stated, and that labels which carry vague terms such as 'lactobacilli' or 'lactic acid-producing bacteria' are not purchased. The named, beneficial probiotic organism(s) should be clearly listed by both their genus and species, for example *Bifidobacterium* (genus) *bifidum* (species) – and not just 'bifidobacteria.'

○ Make sure that there is a statement which guarantees the number of friendly organisms per gram or other measurement (teaspoon, etc.).

○ It is important to see that this number is guaranteed to be the case *at the time of opening the container*, not just at the time of manufacture (the words 'guaranteed shelf-life' will give you this information).

○ The label should say that this number is of 'viable colony-forming units' which means that they are 'whole' organisms and not just fragments of damaged ones.

○ Try never to buy a probiotic which is in tablet form, as this process severely damages the bacteria's potential for colonization.

○ The label should state that the organism is a 'human strain' or 'human-compatible.'

○ To protect the contents the container should (ideally) be made of dark glass.

○ Probiotic products are best taken as powders (dissolved in water) or as a powder in a capsule, and never a liquid or tablet formulation.

○ If possible, ensure that the product also contains some of the supernatant (the culture in which the organism was grown) – as this provides nutrition for the organism. The label will tell you if this is so.

○ Check whether or not the product requires refrigeration after opening – good brands usually do.

○ Ensure that there is an expiry date on the label and that this date has not yet been reached.

○ Probiotic products which are formulated for people who are dairy-sensitive will state clearly what culture medium has been used in their preparation. This may be soya or carrot or some other food base other than a dairy food; if you are allergic to such a product then avoid bacteria grown on it.

GENERAL RULES FOR STORING AND TAKING PROBIOTIC SUPPLEMENTS

○ Probiotic supplements maintain their potency for much longer periods when not exposed to heat or moisture.

○ All probiotic supplements keep best if they are refrigerated.

○ For therapeutic dosages, avoid liquids and gelatin capsules, which have a high moisture content, as this causes the probiotics to lose their potency rapidly – pure powdered freeze-dried bacterial cultures are best.

○ Mix powdered probiotic supplements in unchlorinated, tepid water to help the freeze-dried bacteria to revive and become active again.

○ Gradually build up to therapeutic dosage levels to prevent rapid, sometimes uncomfortable, changes in intestinal ecology which could give you gas.

○ For best results, *L. acidophilus* and *Bifidobacterium bifidum* should be taken on an empty stomach, 30 to 45 minutes before meals.
○ *L. bulgaricus* is best taken with or immediately after meals.

Caution

People with milk intolerance may not be able to use milk-based products. If the condition is a simple lactose intolerance, most people will do very well on a milk-based *L. acidophilus* supplement. The production of lactase as a byproduct of *L. acidophilus* metabolism has actually been shown to be effective in helping lactose intolerance. For more sensitive patients, the use of milk-free *L. acidophilus* supplements for a month or two may improve lactose intolerance enough for them to be able to tolerate a milk-based supplement.

PROTOCOLS FOR ADULTS

(For infant guidelines see Chapter 10.)

If you are taking antibiotics, the following recommendations for probiotic supplementation are recommended during and following your antibiotic treatment:

1 *L. acidophilus*: $^1/_2$ to 1 teaspoon (or at least 1 capsule) 3 times a day before meals.
2 *Bifidobacterium bifidum*: $^1/_2$ to 1 teaspoon (or at least 1 capsule) 3 times a day before meals.
3 If possible, take probiotic supplements and antibiotics at different times of day.
4 Continue supplementation for a month at therapeutic levels (points 1 and 2, above) after finishing the course of antibiotics.

In cases of acute intestinal distress:

○ *L. acidophilus* and *B. bifidum*: 1 teaspoon (or 1 capsule) of both every hour until symptoms cease.

In cases of chronic constipation:

○ *Lactobacillus bulgaricus*: 2 teaspoons (or 2 capsules) 2 to 3 times a day with meals, for several weeks.
○ When the bowels are behaving again, take maintenance dosages (*see page 195*) of *L. acidophilus* and *Bifidobacterium bifidum*.

In cases of infection or to improve white blood cell counts:

○ *L. bulgaricus*: 2 teaspoons (or 2 capsules) 3 to 4 times a day with meals.
○ After two weeks, add 1 teaspoon (or 1 capsule) of both *L. acidophilus* and *Bifidobacterium bifidum* 3 times a day before meals.

In cases of candidiasis (thrush – *see also Chapter 7 for advice on diet and supplements for this condition*):

Oral administration:

○ *L. acidophilus* and *Bifidobacterium bifidum*: 1 teaspoon (or 1 capsule) of each 3 times a day before meals.
○ *L. bulgaricus*: 2 to 3 teaspoons (or 2 to 3 capsules) 3 times a day with meals, for several weeks.
○ If severe Candida die-off symptoms occur (*see Chapter 7*), reduce this dosage and then gradually increase it again.

Local application:

○ Fill two large (size 00) or four small (size 0) gelatin capsules (obtainable from pharmacies) with *L. acidophilus*. Insert vaginally or rectally before bedtime, for 10 days.
○ Alternatively, mix 1 rounded teaspoon of *L. acidophilus* with 2 tablespoons of plain regular yogurt (not low- or non-fat). Insert vaginally or rectally before bedtime, for 10 days.
○ *Note:* Do not fill capsules ahead of time, as the high moisture content of the capsule gelatin may damage the ability of the acidophilus bacteria to colonize.

Douche:

○ Mix 1 teaspoon of *L. acidophilus* in warm water. Stir briskly and let this stand for at least five minutes. Stir again. Use this as a douche each morning for 10 days.

Maintenance dosages:

○ *L. acidophilus*: 1 teaspoon (or 1 capsule) once daily on an empty stomach.
○ *Bifidobacterium bifidum*: $1/4$ teaspoon powder once daily on an empty stomach.

Lacto-vegetarians, athletes and those of African or Asian ancestry may have a need for more *Bifidobacterium* than *L. acidophilus*, due to their high intake of complex carbohydrates (in the case of the first two) or inherited traditional dietary patterns (for the latter two). For such individuals the following is suggested:

○ *Bifidobacterium bifidum*: $3/4$ teaspoon once daily.
○ *L. acidophilus*: $1/2$ teaspoon once daily.

If you *have* to take antibiotics – as well as taking appropriate levels of probiotics (*see above*) plus live yogurt (unless you are allergic to dairy foods), it is suggested that you can lessen the damage caused by the antibiotics by taking the following supplements/herbs during the course and for at least a week after the end of the course:

○ One or other of the herbs which help immune function as discussed in Chapter 6 – in particular Echinacea, if available – 3 500-mg doses at least twice daily during the period of the infection.
○ Vitamin C as discussed in Chapter 6 – between 2 and 10 grams daily to enhance immune function – but be prepared for (harmless) diarrhea. Continue after the infection with at least 2 grams daily for some weeks.
○ Also consider detoxification methods, such as short-term immune-enhancing fasting as discussed in Chapter 5 – but consult a naturopath or suitably qualified nutritional expert for guidance if you are new to fasting.
○ It is important to ensure adequate liquid intake – at least 10 cups of water a day.

When Should You Use Antibiotics?

○ Only if there is an absolute need, and ideally once less aggressive methods have been tried. Avoid echinacea during pregancy.
○ 'Absolute need' means an infection, of bacterial origin, which has the potential to cause further damage – affecting your eyes, ears or chest, for example – and which is not responsive to gentler methods (herbs, fasting, nutrition, etc. as described in Chapter 6).
○ Remember that almost all throat, chest and sinus infections, as well as all flu and colds, are of viral origin and are therefore *totally* unresponsive to antibiotics.

Above all, remember that immune enhancement is possible using nutrition (and possibly herbs or homeopathy) and that reliance on your own immune system is almost always the best option, unless you are immune compromised in some way – in which case why not work to improve this vital defense system by following some of the guidelines in Chapters 5 and 6?

10: Children, Antibiotics, and Probiotics

The Friendly Bacteria Arrive

○ Within a few days of birth, an infant's gastrointestinal tract will have been colonized by friendly bacteria.
○ What happens during the birth influences the pattern of colonization. For example, *Bifidobacterium infantis* was found in around 60 percent of 4- to 6-day-old babies who had been born vaginally, but in only 9 percent of babies born by caesarean section.
○ Whether or not a baby is breastfed also decides what happens in the colonization process. Breastfed babies have a large majority of bifidobacteria, while those who are bottle-fed with infant formula or cow's milk have fewer of these.

The very first milk a breastfed baby receives contains colostrum, which carries in it enormously important immune-enhancing substances that help the baby's defense systems to control (among other things) bacteria such as E. coli, and encourages the colonization of the tract with *Bifidobacterium infantis*.

There is strong evidence that colonization of the infant digestive tract starts via the mouth. Slowly, over the first few days, the bacteria work their way down until all of the intestines are inhabited. These bacteria 'pay their way' by means of the life-preserving and health-enhancing services they offer us.

Infant feed formulations and cow's milk do not contain the essential ingredients of breastmilk.

Why the Change over the Past 25 Years?

The incidence of childhood allergy has increased dramatically over the past 25 years, with conditions such as eczema and asthma now five to six times more prevalent.

An allergy is an excessively violent 'normal' response to an allergen; we need to ask ourselves why the immune systems of children, worldwide, are now over-reacting by as much as 500 to 600 percent compared with a quarter of a century ago.

Explanations are offered by French and German researchers, who have examined two different features:

1 the quality and quantity of friendly bacteria in the intestinal tracts of infants worldwide[2]
2 the quality of breastmilk throughout the world.[3]

By carefully examining the status of thousands of infants today and comparing this with records available from earlier research, French researchers have been able to determine that breastfed babies today have a level of the most useful friendly bacteria very similar to that found in formula (bottle-) fed babies 25 to 30 years ago.

This means that breastfed babies today suffer from the same sorts and levels of allergy and infection that previously affected bottle-fed babies.

Why?

Whereas in the past the dominant strain of the bifido-bacteria in the infant intestine was *Bifidobacterium infantis*, now *Bifidobacterium bifidum* and *Bifidobacterium longum* (which are both adult strains) are predominant. Other changes include the now widespread presence, even in breastfed infant bowels, of undesirable bacteria such as E. coli, Shigella and Clostridium.

This change in the strains which dominate in babies is worldwide and has major health implications aside from the six-fold rise in the incidence of allergies.

For example, E. coli infection is responsible for thousands of infant deaths every year and is commonly involved in cases of uncontrolled diarrhea in infants, as are the bacteria Shigella and Salmonella. These organisms produce extremely toxic substances which are capable of causing damage and even death.

Bifidobacterium infantis, the main (or what should be the main) friendly colonizer of a healthy infant digestive tract, can usually control these dangerous bacteria. But to do so it has to be present and in a good state of health itself.

An army which is not alerted and in position, and which is weaker than it ought to be, can hardly defend the territory which is being invaded. And it can do even less if it has been infiltrated by the enemy, which is virtually what happens when undesirable alien bacteria (E. coli, for example) take up residence in regions where they would normally be excluded, simply because the normal defenses (*Bifidobacterium infantis*, for example) are weakened and inefficient.

What Are the Signs of a Reduction in Bifido-bacterium infantis?

The French researchers[4] reported that 'Breastfeeding induces liquid feces with a "cheesy" odor and a pH [acid level] of around 5.0. The feces of formula-fed infants looks and smells like those of an adult and has a pH of between 6.0 and 7.0 [less acidic than 5.0].'

Natural Alternatives to Antibiotics

WHAT THIS MEANS

○ It means that the normally acid levels of the bowel, which help to control undesirable bacteria, are reduced in formula-fed babies. Unfortunately this change is now also occurring in breastfed babies.
○ There are more potentially harmful E. coli bacteria (and other undesirables) in the digestive tracts of babies fed on formula and cow's milk.
○ It has always been known that formula-fed babies have a far greater chance of developing allergies (and infections) than breastfed babies – and unfortunately, while breastfed babies are still relatively better protected than bottle-fed ones, the gap is narrowing.

The question is, what has happened to reduce the health and efficiency of the friendly bacteria in breastfed babies?

German research suggests that these changes are mainly due to pollution – most notably by substances such as dioxin and various petrochemicals which have found themselves into the water supplies worldwide.

Samples of breastmilk taken from women in all parts of the planet, from all continents and environments – including city dwellers, women living in rural settings, Amazonian jungles, the wastes of Alaska and the South Sea islands – were analyzed with great care. What emerged from this study was the startling fact that relative levels of toxic chemicals such as polychlorinated dibenzo-P-dioxin and polychlorinated dibenzoflurans are now universally present, in high levels, in the breastmilk of every new mother.

WHERE DOES THIS TOXICITY COME FROM?

These toxic chemical environmental pollutants derive from a wide range of sources, including:

○ herbicides such as weed killers – used in gardening and in industrial farming, and therefore present on most vegetables and much fruit
○ wood preservatives – found in every home and most new furniture
○ chemicals used in paper manufacturing – and therefore present in many household paper products
○ garden and farm pesticides – and therefore found on most fruit and vegetables as well as in many animal products such as meat and dairy fats and fish oils (animals, including humans, store toxic materials in their fatty tissues)
○ garbage incineration smoke and byproducts.

The toxic chemicals used and produced in modern industrialized settings have entered the atmosphere and spread worldwide. They have entered the food chain (of plants, animals and humans) and are found in the fatty tissues of everyone on the planet; not surprisingly, therefore, they are found in the milk of almost all animals, including humans.

When consumed by a baby, these toxic substances are capable of seriously damaging the most important of the friendly bacteria, *Bifidobacterium infantis*. This means that infants are in the front line of pollution damage.

Does This Mean That Women Should Not Breastfeed?

Of course not, since even with this toxicity, breastfed babies are infinitely healthier than bottle-fed ones, with less likelihood of acquiring allergy and infection.

The tragedy, which is underlined by the enormous (and growing) rise in allergy rates, is that the health protection which breastfeeding once offered infants has been reduced, although it is still much greater than that provided by alternatives to breastmilk.

Answers

One of the world's leading researchers into probiotics is Professor Rasic of the former Yugoslavia,[5] who believes that all babies should now be supplemented with *B. infantis*. He suggests between 100 million and 1 billion bacteria per day, which is easily achieved using the maintenance dosages listed below. This, he states, 'ensures a steady supply of these friendly bacteria to the intestinal tract which allow these organisms to help the resident organisms to combat harmful bacteria.'

Fortunately the option of being able to supplement babies with uncontaminated friendly bacterial strains (*see below*) does exist – although it is not cheap. If at all possible this is a choice which all parents should consider for the general protection of their infants. These products, which have been specifically formulated and designed for infants, are available from well-stocked health stores and some pharmacies, though you may have to ask for them to be ordered specially.

There is strong evidence to support the idea that babies and young children who have to take antibiotics should have a supplemental replenishment of bacteria (reflorastation) during and after the course of antibiotics.[6] Such supplementation should be automatic every time antibiotics are used, since even a short course of antibiotics will damage the friendly flora.

MAKE SURE YOU GET THE RIGHT PROBIOTIC

Because of their very real physiological differences (when compared with adults), infants must *never* be given adult forms or strains of probiotics such as *L. acidophilus* without the specific recommendation of a physician experienced in probiotics, as these organisms produce too much lactic acid for the delicate infant digestive tract to handle, until such time as they have been weaned on to solid food. An exception is during acute gastroenteritis – see notes below.

PROBIOTIC GUIDELINES FOR INFANTS

Note

Only the forms of bifidobacteria listed in this chapter should be supplemented to young children.

Because there are a number of dubious products on the market, and because the area of probiotic supplementation is relatively new, you are strongly advised to follow the advice offered below, which is based on the experience of many years of clinical practice and the research of numerous experts.[7]

Whenever purchasing a probiotic product for a child, ensure the following:

- The product contains only one organism – not a cocktail.
- The organism is meant for infants (*see below*) and that this is clearly stated on the container.
- The organism is a 'human strain.'
- The container is (ideally) made of dark glass.
- The product is a powder and not in liquid, capsule or tablet form.
- If possible, the product should also contain some of the supernatant (the culture in which the organism was grown) – as this provides nutrition for the organism.
- There is a statement as to the number of organisms per gram or other measurement (teaspoon, etc.).
- This number is guaranteed to be the case *at the time of opening* and not just at the time of manufacture of the product ('guaranteed shelf-life').
- This number should be of 'viable colony-forming units.'
- The product requires refrigeration after opening.
- There is an expiry date and that the product is within that time limit.
- Products designed for those who are dairy sensitive state clearly what culture medium has been used in their production.

Infants:

○ Freeze-dried powders made up of billions of living but temporarily inactivated friendly bacteria may be mixed in a small amount of water and administered by dropper, thoroughly mixed with formula or a juice.
○ In infants the gastric acid is mild enough not to be a consideration, so that although when adults take acidophilus and bifidus bacteria they commonly do so at a time well away from mealtimes to protect the bacteria from being digested, with infants this does not apply.

Toddlers:

○ The freeze-dried probiotic powders should be given on an empty stomach, if at all possible – in a lukewarm drink (water, juice); 15–30 minutes before meals is generally the best time to recommend.

DURING AND FOLLOWING A COURSE OF ANTIBIOTICS

When antibiotics are being taken, probiotics should be taken at least 3 times daily, at separate times from the antibiotics. This should continue for at least one month after the end of the antibiotic course.

○ Infants: $^{1}/_{8}$ teaspoon *Bifidobacterium infantis*, 3 times a day.
○ Toddlers: $^{1}/_{4}$ teaspoon *Bifidobacterium infantis*, 3 times a day.
○ Continue supplementation for a month at these therapeutic levels, even after stopping the course of antibiotics.
○ Follow this by giving maintenance dosages (*see below*).

Acute intestinal distress in infants – such as gastroenteritis:

○ $^{1}/_{8}$ to $^{1}/_{4}$ teaspoon of both *L. acidophilus* and *Bifidobacterium infantis* every hour until symptoms cease.

Maintenance dosages:

○ Infants: $^1/_8$ to $^1/_4$ teaspoon of *Bifidobacterium infantis*, once daily.
○ Toddlers: $^1/_4$ to $^1/_2$ teaspoon of *Bifidobacterium infantis*, once daily, on an empty stomach, if possible.

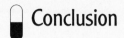 Conclusion

Antibiotics, correctly used, in the right situations, save lives.

This book has aimed to explain how and why antibiotics have been, and often continue to be, used wrongly, and the horrifying consequences this can produce. It is a plea for the correct, selective, safe use of antibiotics when they are really needed.

Throughout this book I have tried to offer specific advice and information for people who have to – appropriately – take antibiotics, so that the negative effects can be minimized.

A voice of protest must be raised against the ominous, almost complete inaction on the part of officialdom, most members of the medical profession, the farming industry and food producers in general (excepting organic growers, of course), the media and, above all, the general public – the consumers of antibiotics either as drugs or in their food, who in the end hold the power to influence both official policy and the media by their actions and beliefs.

The (over)use of drugs designed to control disease-causing microorganisms is producing resistant strains, so leading to the emergence of diseases which can no longer be controlled.

We can no longer expect to be able to force antibiotics into animals (diseased in the first place because of the unnatural ways in which they are bred for slaughter, or in order to speed up their growth) and then eat these animals without seriously harming ourselves.

We can no longer use antibiotics in the treatment of human disease in ways which are guaranteed to result in resistant strains – superbugs – without this actually happening.

Not only have we managed to produce an environment in which superbugs have evolved, but knowing that we have done so we continue to do so.

The heroes meant to save us – antibiotics – turn out to be working for the enemy by making it stronger and weakening our natural defenses. Some bacterial strains have evolved which are quite simply resistant to all antibiotics, while others have learned remarkable ways in which to 'hide' from the drugs which should be able to kill them.

Looking at this doomsday scenario – of increasingly powerful drugs being used to kill ever more powerful disease-causing bacteria – and so leading to the development of even more resistance – may seem to leave no room for maneuver. However, somewhere in this problem lies a seed of hope: we *can* do something about it.

It is important to note that while the development of superbugs represents one major negative effect of the use and misuse of antibiotics, it is certainly not the only one. Most antibiotics seriously damage the friendly bacteria that live in us, and this damage can – in a major way – contribute to:

○ high cholesterol
○ menopausal symptoms
○ premenstrual symptoms
○ gynecological problems
○ liver disease
○ chronic digestive and bowel problems
○ increased risk of bladder infections
○ serious arthritic conditions
○ and depressed immune function.

Where Does the Blame Lie?[1,2,3]

○ There has been a failure on the part of health authorities, both local and national, to appreciate the documented evidence linking antibiotic use and health problems.

○ Health care professionals have prescribed and delivered antibiotics inappropriately. Their own professional journals have been hinting to them for years, and lately telling them unequivocally, that there are conditions for which antibiotics are useless and undesirable. Yet prescribing continues at increasing rates.

○ Many doctors prescribe antibiotics 'just in case' when there is overwhelming evidence that the only time they should be prescribed is when a bacterial infection has been identified, and even then, that only the correct antibiotic should be selected.

○ Many doctors and dentists give broad-spectrum antibiotics, before surgery or dental extractions, for example, in order to prevent infection – or so they think. The evidence is that no benefit is gained from such practices, which add enormously to the chances of bacteria developing resistance and which cause enormous damage to the normal 'friendly' flora living in and on the person, with the possibility that these changes will lead to further health problems sooner or later.

○ The 'just in case' approach in which a prophylactic ('preventive') dose is prescribed – often excessively used before caesarean section, for example – leads to no benefit to the patient, and even possible harm. As leading American researcher Dr. Marc Lappe puts it, 'Such over-treatment comes close to professional irresponsibility.'[4]

○ Apart from occasional TV documentaries and newspaper and magazine feature articles, the media largely ignores this story – possibly because of editorial pressure relating to the advertising power of the pharmaceutical companies, whose profits largely depend upon continued sales of these drugs. Courageous – and persistent – journalism is required to lay the options clearly before the public.

○ Government organs have failed to tackle either the medical overuse of antibiotics or the food industry and farming misuse and abuse of antibiotics in food production. The reasons for such inaction probably lie somewhere between ignorance and arrogance – much the same area which allowed the use in food production of ground-up sheep parts in the feed of vegetarian cows – with the end result we all now face: BSE (in its animal and, increasingly, its human form – vCJD).

○ Consumers – ourselves – have accepted the cheap food production and the quick-fix drug route to health, despite warnings over the past 25 years by ecologists and activists, usually branded as cranks and quacks. We have accepted the cheapness of food and the rapid exit from the sickbed in blissful ignorance of the fact that there are consequences to such actions which cannot be evaded forever. If we subvert natural processes we reap a rotten harvest:

> ○ If we feed minced-up sheep to cows, then something unpredictable – but predictably undesirable – will happen.
> ○ Put antibiotics into chicken feed, and you get eggs with high levels of resistant food-poisoning potential.
> ○ Use antibiotics to kill the bacteria involved in infections which the healthy immune system can easily handle, and you end up with resistant organisms and a damaged immune system.
> ○ Pump antibiotics into children for conditions not even caused by bacteria, 'just in case' of secondary bacterial infection, and in time recurrent bacterial, or viral, or yeast infections will evolve in a weakened immune system.
> ○ Overuse antibiotics and the seeds are sown for massive untreatable infectious epidemics in the future.

Natural Alternatives to Antibiotics

We have been warned, we have seen the signs: the doom-laden headlines about superbugs, the return of TB – and yet we and our doctors seem to march headlong toward the abyss, cheerfully hopeful that somehow science (which got us into this mess) will save us.

Unlike some predictions of imminent worldwide catastrophe, such as the periodic forecasts relating to greenhouse effects, global warming, ozone layer destruction – which we can worry about but do little to alter. However, the fact that there are indeed things that we as individuals can do about many of these dangers offers hope in what is otherwise a gloomy story. We can, individually, make decisions which will alter how the antibiotic onslaught affects us:

○ We can enhance our immune systems.
○ We can resist antibiotics unless essential – by learning more about health, disease and infection, and speaking to our medical advisers about the risks and alternatives involved.
○ We can learn to reverse some of the inevitable internal ecological damage which antibiotics cause, should we absolutely have to take them – and there may be times that we do.
○ We can avoid – absolutely – food containing antibiotics, by refusing to buy or eat farmed fish and anything but organic, free-range meats, poultry and dairy products.

The harvest we have sown is now being reaped. We can choose to ignore the dangers ahead or to do something about them. This is the choice we face and the hope that is offered in this book.

References

CHAPTER 1

1. Hall, C. 'Infections kill 5000 a year in hospitals', *Daily Telegraph* [London], 17th September 1997: page 5
2. Radestky, P. 'Killer Hospitals', *Longevity* (July 1994): page 18
3. Report in the *Daily Telegraph* by Roger Highfield, Science Editor, 6th August 1997: page 10
4. O'Grady, F., Lambert, H., Finch, R., Greenwood, D. (eds). *Antibiotic and Chemotherapy* (7th edn; NY: Churchill Livingstone, 1997)
5. Wick, A. 'The eczema X factor' *Telegraph Magazine* 13th September 1997: page 63
6. O'Grady *et al.*, op cit: page 786
7. *Daily Telegraph*, 6th August 1997, op cit.
8. McKenna, J. *Alternatives to Antibiotics* (Dublin: Gill & Macmillan, 1996)
9. Report in the *Times* [London] by Jeremy Laurance, Health Correspondent, 7th March 1997.
10. Diamant, M. and Diamant, D. 'Abuse and timing of use of antibiotics in acute otitis media', *Archives of Otorhynolaryngology* 100.3 (September 1974): pages 226–34
11. van Buchen, F. *et al.* 'Therapy of acute otitis media: Meryngotomy, antibiotics, or neither?', *Lancet* 2 (1981): pages 883–7
12. Cantekin, E. *et al.* 'Antimicrobial therapy for otitis media with effusion', *Journal of the American Medical Association* 266.23 (December 18 1991): pages 3309–17
13. van Buchen, F. *et al.* 'Acute otitis media: a new treatment strategy', *British Medical Journal* 290 (1985): pages 1033–7

14. French, G. and Phillips, I., in O'Grady *et al.* op cit.
15. Ibid.
16. Irwin, A. 'Ventilation tests "miss dormant bugs'"; report in *Daily Telegraph*, 17th September 1997: page 5

CHAPTER 2

1. Carlson, E. 'Enhancement by Candida of S. aureus, S. marcescens, S. faecalis in the establishment of infection', *Infection and Immunity* 39.1 (1983): pages 193–7
2. French, G. and Phillips, I., in O'Grady, F., Lambert, H., Finch, R., Greenwood, D. (eds). *Antibiotic and Chemotherapy* (7th edn; NY: Churchill Livingstone, 1997)
3. *Food Magazine* Jan/Mar 1996
4. Lappe, M. *When Antibiotics Fail* (Berkeley, CA: North Atlantic Press, 1995)

CHAPTER 3

1. Lacey, R., in Cannon, G. *Superbugs* (London: Virgin, 1995)
2. Warner, E. (ed). *Savills System of Clinical Medicine* (14th edn; London: Edward Arnold, 1964)
3. Hughes, D., in O'Grady F., Lambert, H., Finch, R., Greenwood, D. (eds). *Antibiotic and Chemotherapy* (7th edn; NY: Churchill Livingstone, 1997; chapter 34 – Sulphonamides)
4. Rowley, N. *Basic Clinical Science* (London: Hodder & Stoughton, 1991)
5. Garrod, L., in O'Grady *et al.*, op cit. (chapter 1 – Historical introduction)
6. Lappe, M. *When Antibiotics Fail* (Berkeley, CA: North Atlantic Press, 1995)
7. Henry, J. *British Medical Association's New Guide to Medicines and Drugs* (London: Dorling Kindersley, 1995)
8. Cannon, *Superbugs* op cit.
9. Pizzorno, J. *10 Drugs I Would Never Use* (Brookline, MA: Natural Health, 1997)

10. Garrod, op cit.

CHAPTER 4

1. Morton, I. (ed). *Antibiotics – the comprehensive guide* (London: Bloomsbury, 1990)
2. Henry, J. *British Medical Association's New Guide to Medicines and Drugs* (London: Dorling Kindersley, 1995)
3. Cannon, G. *Superbugs* (London: Virgin, 1995)
4. Lappe, M. *When Antibiotics Fail* (Berkeley, CA: North Atlantic Press, 1995)
5. O'Grady, F., Lambert, H., Finch, R., Greenwood, D. (eds). *Antibiotic and Chemotherapy* (7th edn; NY: Churchill Livingstone, 1997)
6. Greenwood, D., in O'Grady *et al.*, op cit. (chapter 1 – Historical introduction)
7. Gemmel, C., in O'Grady *et al.*, op cit. (chapter 8 – Antibiotics and the immune system)
8. Information derived mainly from references 1, 2 and 5.
9. Ibid.
10. Ibid.
11. Ibid.
12. Gemmel, op cit.
13. Information derived mainly from references 1, 2 and 5.
14. Ibid.
15. Gemmel, op cit.
16. Information derived mainly from references 1, 2 and 5.
17. Ibid.
18. Ibid.
19. Ball, A., in O'Grady *et al.*, op cit. (chapter 7 – Antibiotic toxicity)

CHAPTER 5

1. Selye, H. *The Stress of Life* (New York: McGraw Hill, 1976)
2. Ngu, V. 'Fever: Thermodynamics applied to the leucocyte', *Medical Hypothesis* 33 (1991): pages 241–4

3. Pizzorno, J. *Total Wellness – improve your health by understanding the body's healing systems* (Rocklin, CA:. Prima, 1996)

4. Standish, L. 'One-year open trial of naturopathic treatment of HIV infection (HARP) study', *Journal of Naturopathic Medicine* 3.1 (1992): pages 42–64

5. Ettinger, N. *et al.* 'Respiratory Effects of Smoking Cocaine', *American Journal of Medicine* 87 (1989): page 664

6. Flaws, B. *Nine Ounces: A nine-part program for the prevention of AIDS in HIV+ persons* (Boulder, CO: Blue Poppy Press, 1989)

7. Chaitow, L. *Body-Mind Purification Program* (Simon and Schuster, 1989)

8. Ibid.

9. Cousins, N. *Anatomy of an Illness* (Bantam, 1987)

10. Newman, Turner R. *Naturopathic Medicine* (Thorsons, 1990)

11. *AIDS 1990 – A Physicians' Manual* (Laurel, MD: Life Science Universal Inc., 1990)

12. Simonton, C. *Getting Well Again* (Bantam, 1986)

13. Solomon, G. *Psychoneuroimmunology* (Academic Press, 1981)

14. Standish, op cit.

15. Quoted in Chaitow, L. and Martin, S. *World Without AIDS* (Thorsons, 1989)

16. 'Depression, stress and immunity', *Lancet* (27th June 1987): pages 1487–8

17. Chaitow, L. *The Stress Protection Plan* (Thorsons, 1991)

18. Uden, A. *et al.* 'Neutrophil function and clinical performance after total fasting in patients with rheumatoid arthritis', *Annals of Rheumatic Diseases* 42 (1983): pages 45–51

CHAPTER 6

1. Williams, R. *Biochemical Individuality* (Austin, TX: University of Texas Press, 1982)

2. Standish, L. 'One-year open trial of naturopathic treatment of HIV infection (HARP) study', *Journal of Naturopathic Medicine* 3.1 (1992): pages 42–64

3. Sanchez, A. *et al.* 'Role of sugars in human neutrophilic phagocytosis', *America Journal of Clinical Nutrition* 26.11 (1973): pages 1180–4

4. Mertin, J. 'Essential fatty acid and Cell-Mediated immunity', *Prog. Lipid Research* 20 (1981): pages 851–6

5. Chaitow, L. *Stone Age Diet* (Macdonald Optima, 1987)

6. Brayton, R. *et al.* 'Effects of alcohol on leucocyte mobilization etc.', *New England Journal of Medicine* 282.3 (1970): pages 123–8; Saxena, A. *et al.* 'Immunomodulating effect of caffeine', *Indian Journal of Experimental Biology* 22.6 (1984): pages 293–301

7. McGovern Senate Committee on Nutrition: Guidelines; NACNE Dietary recommendations UK 1986

8. Standish, op cit

9. Brayton, op cit

10. Huang, C. *et al.* 'Nutritional status of patients with AIDS', *Clinical Chemistry* 34.10 (1988): pages 1957–9

11. Palmblad, J. 'Malnutrition associated immune deficiency syndrome', *Acta Med Scand* 222 (1987): pages 1–3

12. Mantera-Tienza, E. *et al.* 'Low vitamin B_6 in HIV infection', *Fifth International Conference on AIDS* (Montreal, June, 1989): page 468

13. Herbert, V. 'Vitamin B_{12}, folate and lithium in AIDS' (Abstract), *Clinical Research* 37.2 (1989): page 594A

14. Harriman, G. *et al.* 'Vitamin B_{12} malabsorption in AIDS', *Archives Internal Medicine* 149 (1989): pages 2039–41

15. Dworkin, B. *et al.* 'Selenium deficiency in AIDS', *Journal of Parenteral and Enteral Nutrition* 10.4 (1986): pages 405–7

16. Fabris, N. *et al.* 'AIDS, zinc deficiency and thymic hormone failure', *Journal of American Medical Association* 259 (1988): pages 839–40

17. Pulse, T. *et al.* 'A significant improvement in a clinical pilot study utilizing nutritional supplements, essential fatty acids and stabilized aloe vera juice in 29 HIV seropositive, ARC and AIDS patients', *Journal for the Advancement of Medicine* 3.4 (1990): pages 209–30

18. Rheinhardt, A. *et al.* 'Mechanisms of viricidal activity of retinoids', *Antimicrobial Agents Chemotherapy* 17.6 (1980): pages 1034–7

19. Dolbeare, F. *et al.* 'Beta-carotene – an unusual type of lipid antioxidant', *Science* 224 (1984): pages 569–73

20. Alexander, M. *et al.* 'Oral beta-carotene can increase number of OKT4+ cells in human blood', *Immunology* (letters) 9.4 (1985): pages 221–4

21. Guitierrez, P. 'Influence of ascorbic acid on free radical metabolism of xenobiotics', *Drug Metabolism Review* 18.3/4 (1989): pages 319–43

22. Blakeslee, J., op cit.

23. Bouras, P. *et al.* 'Monocyte locomotion – in vivo effect of ascorbic acid', *Immunopharmacology and Immunotoxicology* 11.1 (1989): pages 119–29

24. Harakeh, S. *et al.* 'Suppression of HIV replication by ascorbate', *Proceedings of National Academy of Sciences* 87 (1990): pages 7245–9

25. Blakeslee, J. *et al.* 'Human T-cell leukaemia virus induction inhibited by retinoids, L-ascorbic acid and DL-alpha tocopherol', *Cancer Research* 45 (1985): pages 3471–6

26. Schwerdt, P. and Schwerdt, C. 'Effect of ascorbic acid on rhinovirus replication', *Proc.Soc.Exp.Biol.Med* 148.4 (1975): pages 1237–43

27. Beisel, W. *et al.* 'Single nutrient effects on immunological functions', *Journal of the American Medical Association* 245.1 (1981): pages 53–8

28. Chaitow, L. and Martin, S. *World Without AIDS* (Thorsons, 1989)

29. Mann, C. 'Vitamin C KOs HIV in QQQ' (UK) 1991

30. Davies, S. and Stewart, A. *Nutritional Medicine* (London: Pan Books, 1987)

31. *AIDS 1990 – A Physicians' Manual* (Laurel, MD: Life Science Universal Inc., 1990)

32. Chaitow and Martin, op cit.

33. *AIDS 1990*, op cit.

34. Falutz, J. *et al.* 'Zinc as cofactor in HIV-induced immunosuppression', *Journal of the American Medical Association* 259.19 (1989): pages 1881–2

35. Erdmann, R. PhD. 'AIDS re-examined', *Felmore Newsletter* (UK), 1987

36. Chaitow, L. and Trenev, N. *Probiotics* (Thorsons, 1989)

37. Weiner, M. *Maximum Immunity* (Gateway Books, 1986)

38. *AIDS 1990*, op cit.

39. *AIDS 1990*, op cit.

40. Pizzorno, J. and Murray, M. *Textbook of Natural medicine* (Bastyr Publications, 1989)

41. Adetumbi, M. *et al.* 'Allium sativum, a natural antibiotic', *Medical Hypothesis* 12 (1983): pages 227–37

42. Vahora, S. *et al.* 'Medicinal use of Indian vegetables', *Planta Medica* 23 (1973): pages 381–93

43. 'Garlic in cryptococcal meningitis' *Chinese Medical Journal* 93 (1980): pages 123–6

44. Sun, Y. *et al.* 'Preliminary observation on the effects of Chinese herbs', *Journal of Biological Response Modifiers* 2 (1983): pages 227–37

45. Sun, Y. *et al.* 'Immune restoration and/or augmentation of local versus host reaction by traditional Chinese herbs', *Cancer* 52.1 (1983): pages 70–3

46. Walker, M. 'Carnivora Therapy in cancer and AIDS', *Explore* 3.5 (1992): pages 10–15

47. Walker, M. 'Carnivora and AIDS', *Townsend Letter for Doctors* (May 1992)

48. Walker, M. 'Carnivora Therapy', *Raum & Zeit* 4.2 (1991)

49. Stimpel, M. *et al.* 'Macrophage activation and induction of cytotoxicity by purified polysaccharide fractions from Echinacea purpurea', *Infection and Immunity* 46 (1984): pages 845–9

50. Wacker, A. *et al.* 'Virus inhibition by Echinacea purpurea', *Planta Medica* 33 (1978): pages 89–102

51. Brekhmann, E. *Man and Biologically Active Substances* (London: Pergamon Press, 1980)

52. Takada, A. *et al.* 'Restoration of radiation injury by Ginseng', *Journal of Radiation* 22 (1981): pages 323–5

53. Abe, N. *et al.* 'Interferon induction by Glycyrrhizin', *Microbiology and Immunology* 26.6 (1982): pages 535–9

54. Mischer, L. *et al.* 'Antimicrobial agents from higher plants', *Journal of Natural Products* 43.2 (1980): pages 259–69

55. Kiso, Y. *et al.* 'Mechanism of antihepatotoxic activity of glycyrrhizin', *Planta Medica* 50.4 (1984): pages 298–302

56. Juroyanagi, T. *et al.* 'Effect of prednisone and glycyrrhizin on passive transfer of experimental allergic encephalomyitis', *Allergy* 15 (1966): pages 670–5

57. Onuchi, K. 'Glycyrrhizin inhibits prostaglandin E2 production', *Prostaglandins in Medicine* 7.5 (1981): pages 457–63

58. Kumazai, A. *et al.* 'Effects of glycyrrhizin on thymolytic and immunosuppressive action of cortisone', *Endocrinology Japan* 14,1 (1967): pages 39–42

59. Abe, N. *et al.*, op cit.

60. Pompei, R. *et al.* 'Glycyrrhizic acid inhibits virus growth and inactivates virus particles', *Nature* 281 (1979): pages 689–90

61. Ito, M. *et al.* 'Mechanism of inhibitory effect of Glycyrrhizin on replication of HIV', *Antiviral Research* 10 (1988): pages 289–98

62. Sharma, R. *et al.* 'Berberine tannate in acute diarrhoea', *Indian Pediatric Journal* 7 (1978): pages 496–502

63. Choudray, V. *et al.* 'Berberine in Giardiasis', Indian Pediatrics 9: pages 143–146 1972

64. Sack, R. *et al.* 'Berberine inhibits intestinal secretory response of Vibrio cholerae, E.Coli enterotoxins', *Infection and Immunity* 35.2 (1982): pages 471–5

65. Meruelo, D. *et al.* 'Therapeutic agents with dramatic retroviral activity', *Proceedings of National Academy of Sciences* 85 (1988): pages 5230–4

66. Someya, H. 'Effect of a constituent of hypericum on infection and multiplication of Epstein Barr virus', *Journal of Tokyo Medical College* 43.5 (1985): pages 815–26

67. Barbagallo, C. *et al.* 'Antimicrobial activity of three Hypericum species', *Fitoteripia* LVIII.3 (1987): pages 175–7

68. 'Information on Medical Science and Technology', *Guangdong Institute of Medicine and Health* 8–9 (1973): page 33

69. Report in *Daily Telegraph* by Roger Highfield, Science Editor, 6th August 1997: page 10

70. Wagner, H. and Prokcsh, A. 'Immunostimulating drugs from fungi and higher plants', in *Progress in Medicinal and Economic Plant Research* (vol 1; London: Academic Press, 1983)

71. Maughan, R. *et al.* 'Effects of pollen extract upon adolescent swimmers', *British Journal of Sports Medicine* 16.3 (1982): pages 142–5

72. *Foundations of Chinese Herb Prescribing* (Long Beach, CA: Oriental Healing Arts Institute)

73. Pizzorno and Murray, op cit.

74. Neville, A. *et al.* 'Whole body hyperthermia induces interleukin-1 in vivo', *Lymphokine Research* 7.3 (1988): pages 201–5; Park, M. *et al.* 'Effect of whole body hyperthermia on immune cell activity of cancer patients', *Lymphokine Research* 9.2 (1990): pages 213–21

75. Martin, L. *et al.* 'Disinfection and inactivation of human T-lymphotrophic virus-111 lymphadenopathy-associated virus', *Journal of Infectious Disease* 152.2 (1985): pages 300–403

76. Sminia, P. *et al.* 'What is a safe heat dose which can be applied to normal brain tissue?', *International Journal of Hyperthermia* 5.1 (1989): pages 115–17

77. Standish, op cit

78. Tyrrell, D., Barrow, I. and Arthur, J. 'Local hyperthermia benefits natural and experimental common colds', *British Medical Journal* 298 (1989): pages 1280–3

79. Spire, B., Dormont, D., Barre-Sinoussi, F. *et al.* 'Inactivation of lymphadenopathy-associated virus by heat, gamma rays, and ultraviolet light', *The Lancet* 1.8422 (January 26, 1985): pages 188–9

80. Thrash, Agatha, MD, and Calvin, MD. *Home Remedies* (Seale, AL: Thrash Publications, 1981): page 124

81. Standish, op cit

82. Weatherburn, H. 'Hyperthermia and AIDS Treatment', *British Journal of Radiology* 61.729 (September, 1988): page 862

83. Sawtell, N. M. and Thompson, R. L. 'Rapid In Vivo Reactivation of Herpes Simplex Virus in Latently Infected Murine Ganglionic Neurons after Transient Hyperthermia', *Journal of Virology* 66.4 (April, 1992): pages 2150–6

84. Skibba, J. L., Powers, R. H. *et al.* 'Oxidative stress as a precursor to the irreversible hepatocellular injury caused by hyperthermia', *International Journal Hyperthermia* 7.5 (1991): pages 749–61

85. Tyrrell, Barrow and Arthur, op cit.

86. Ernst, E. 'Hydrotherapy research', *Physiotherapy* 76.4: pages 207–10
87. Cracium, T. *et al.* 'Neurohumoral modification after acupuncture', *American Journal of Acupuncture* 21 (1973): page 67
88. Tykochinskaia, E. 'Acupuncture as a method of reflex therapy', *Veprosy Psikhatrii I Nerripathologii* 7 (1960): pages 249–60
89. Yang, C. 'Clinical Report Sansi Acupuncture Symposium', reported in Wensall, L. MD. *Acupuncture in Medical Practice* (Reston Publishing, 1980)
90. Smith, M. and Rabinowitz, N. 'Acupuncture Treatment of AIDS', Lincoln Hospital Acupuncture Clinic, March 1985

CHAPTER 7

1. Truss, C. O. *The Missing Diagnosis* (Birmingham, AL: 1982)
2. Brown, R. *AIDS, Cancer and the Medical Establishment* (Robert Spelling, 1986)
3. Crooke, W. *The Yeast Connection* (Professional Books, 1983)
4. Tyson and Associates, 'Protocol for mucocutanous candidiasis (Santa Monica, CA: 1987)
5. Chaitow, L. *Candida Albicans* (Vermont: Healing Arts Press, 1989)
6. Stretch, C. 'Clinical manifestations of HIV infection in women', *Journal of Naturopathic Medicine* 3.1 (1992): pages 12–19
7. Carlson, E. 'Enhancement by Candida of S. aureus, S. marcescens, S. faecalis in the establishment of infection', *Infection and Immunity* 39.1 (1983): pages 193–7
8. The information reported on regarding Dr. Jessop derives from the *Fibromyalgia Network Newsletter* October 1990 through January 1992 Compendium #2, January 1993, May 1993 Compendium, January 1994, July 1994
9. Anthony, H., Birtwistle, S., Eaton, K., Maberly, J. *Environmental Medicines in Clinical Practice*
10. Chaitow, L. and Trenev, N. *Probiotics* (Thorsons, 1989)

CHAPTER 8

1. Muting, D. *et al.* 'The effect of bacterium bifidum on intestinal Bacterial flora and toxic protein metabolites in chronic liver disease', *American Journal of Proctology* 19 (1968): pages 336–42
2. Rasic, J. and Kurmann, J. *Bifidobacteria and Their Role* (Boston, MA: Birkhauser Verlag, 1983)
3. Lappe, M. *When Antibiotics Fail* (Berkeley, CA: North Atlantic Press, 1995)
4. Hepner, B. *et al.* 'Hypocholesterolemic effect of yogurt', *American Journal of Clinical Nutrition* 32 (1979): pages 19–24
5. Shahani, K. 'Nutritional and therapeutic aspects of lactobacilli', *Journal of Applied Nutrition* 37.2 (June 1973): pages 136–65
6. Gilliland, S. *et al.* 'Assimilation of cholesterol by L. acidophilus', *Applied and Environmental Microbiology* (February 1985): pages 377–81
7. Simon, G., Gorbach, S., in Leonard Johnson (ed). *Physiology of the GastroIntestinal Tract* (New York: Raven Press, 1981) (chapter 55 – Intestinal Flora in Health and Disease)
8. Eriksson, H. 'Excretion of steroid hormones in adults', *European Journal of Biochemistry* 18 (1971): pages 146–50
9. Ebringer, A. 'The relationship between klebsiella infection and ankylosing spondylitis', *Ballier's Clinical Rheumatology* (1989); Ebringer, A. 'Antibodies to Proteus in rheumatoid arthritis', *Lancet* ii (1985): pages 305–7; Ebringer, A. *et al.* 'Rheumatoid arthritis and proteus – a possible aetiological association', *Rheumatol international* 9 (1989): pages 223–8
10. Jameson, R. 'The prevention of recurrent urinary tract infection in women' *The Practitioner* 216 (Feb 1976): pages 178–81
11. Avorn, J. *et al.* 'Reduction in bacteriuria and pyuria after ingestion of cranberry juice', *Journal of the American Medical Association* 2.1 (1994): pages 45–7
12. Ofek, I. *et al.* 'Anti-escherichia adhesion activity of cranberry and blueberry juices', *New England Journal of Medicine* 324 (1991): page 1599
13. Huwez, F., Thirlwell, D., Cockayne, A., Ala-Aldeen, D. 'Mastic

gum kills *Helicobacter pylori'*, *New England Journal of Medicine* 339 (26) (1998): page 1946.

14. Lauk, L. *et al.* 'In vitro antimicrobial activity of *Pistacia lentiscus L.* extracts: preliminary report', *Journal of Chemotherapy* 8 (1996): pages 207–9.

CHAPTER 9

1. Sneath, P. *Bergey's Manual of Systematic Bacteriology* (vol 2; Baltimore, MD: Williams & Wilkins, 1986)

2. Professor J. Rasic, in Chaitow, L. and Trenev, N. *Probiotics* (London: Thorsons, 1989)

3. Dubos, R. and Schaedler, R. 'Some biological effects of the digestive flora', *American Journal of Medical Sciences* (September 1962): pages 265–71

4. Gilliland, S. *et al.* 'Assimilation of cholesterol by L. acidophilus', *Applied and Environmental Microbiology* (February 1985): pages 377–81

5. Gilliland, S. and Speck, M. 'Antagonistic action of L. acidophilus towards intestinal and food borne pathogens', *Journal of Food Protection* 40 (1977): pages 820–3

6. Friend, B. and Shahani, K. 'Nutritional and therapeutic aspects of lactobacilli', *Journal of Applied Nutrition* 36 (1984): pages 125–53

7. Donovan, P. 'Bowel toxaemia, permeability and disease', in Pizzorno and Murray (eds). *Textbook of Natural Medicine* (Seattle, WA: JBCNM, 1986)

8. Grutte, F. *et al. Human Gastrointestinal Microflora* (Leipzig: JA Barth Verlag, 1980)

9. Savage, D. 'Factors influencing biocontrol of bacterial pathogens in the intestines', *Food Technology* (July 1987): pages 82–7

10. Speck, M. 'Interactions among lactobacilli and man', *Journal of Dairy Sciences* 59 (1975): pages 338–43

11. Dubos and Schaedler, op cit.

CHAPTER 10

1. Rasic, J. and Kurrman, J. *Bifidobacteria and Their Role* (Boston, MA: Birkhauser Verlag, 1983)
2. Beerens, H. *et al.* 'Influence of breastfeeding on bifido flora of the newborn intestine', *American Journal of Clinical Nutrition* 33 (1980): pages 2434–9
3. Schecter, A. *et al.* 'PCDD and PCDF in human milk from Vietnam compared with cow's milk from the North American continent', *Chemosphere* 16 (1987): pages 2003–16; Schecter, A. and Gasiewicz, T. 'Health hazard assessment of chlorinated dioxins and dibenzoflurans contained in human milk', *Chemosphere* 16 (1987): pages 2147–54; Schecter, A. and Gasiewicz, T. *Solving Hazardous Waste Problems* (chapter 12 – 'Human breastmilk levels of dioxins and dibenzoflurans'; American Chemical Society, Washington DC 1987)
4. Beerens, H. *et al.*, op cit.
5. Rasic and Kurrman, op cit.
6. Chaitow, L. and Trenev, N. *Probiotics* (London: Thorsons, 1989)
7. Chaitow and Trenev, op cit; *Probiotic Training Manual* (Natren of California, 1993)

CONCLUSION

1. McTaggart, L. *What Doctors Don't Tell You* (London: Thorsons 1996)
2. Cannon, G. *Superbug* (London: Virgin, 1995)
3. Pizzorno, J. *Total Wellness – improve your health by understanding the body's healing systems* (Rocklin, CA: Prima, 1996)
4. Lappe, M. *When Antibiotics Fail* (Berkeley, CA: North Atlantic Press, 1995)

Index

acidophilus *see Lactobacillus
  acidophilus*
acinetobacter spp 37
acne 169-72, 187
acrosoxacin 79
acupuncture 102, 109, 150-2
AIDS *see* HIV
alcohol:
  in bloodstream 158
  in diet 97-8, 106, 163, 165
allergic reactions 85, 98
allergies 187
  childhood 199
Allium sativum 134
Aloe vera juice 163
Altman, Prof. Sidney 11
amino acid supplementation 165
aminoglycosides 36, 66-9
  side-effects 84, 86
amoxycillin 36, 61, 63, 154
ampicillin 6, 34, 35, 61, 82
androgens, recycling 175
animal farming, use in 17, 21, 23,
  36, 207
    meat as human transfer
      medium 36, 210

residues in food 41, 190, 211
ankylosing spondylitis 175-7, 187
antibacterial drugs 56-7
antibiotics, types 44-50
antifungal treatment:
  complementary 163-6
  drugs 162-3
antigen-specific B-lymphocytes 94
antigens 94
antioxidants 103, 104, 105
antiseptics 56
aplastic anemia 47, 83
asthma 199
Astragalus membranaceus 134
Aureomycin 47, 157
autoimmune conditions 175-7,
  187
azithromycin 75
azlocillin 62

B-lymphocytes (B-cells) 94, 96
bactericidal action 57
bacteriostatic action 57
Ball, Dr. A. 82
Baltimore, Prof. Robert 6
'bamboo spine' 176

Irritable Bowel Syndrome 188
Isatis 137
isoniazid 83
itraconazole 162

Jessop, Dr. Carol 160-2, 167, 169, 174
Joiner-Bey, Dr. Herb 108
joint problems 85

Kakkar, Dr. Vijay 143
kanamycin 155
kidney problems 86
Klebsiella 35-6, 176, 187

Lacey, Prof. Richard 41
Lactobacillus, complete destruction 155
L. acidophilus 25-6, 183
  dosages 193-5, 203, 205
  and lactose intolerance 193
  mutation 52
  supplementation 113, 117, 163, 165
L. brevis 29, 184
L. bulgaricus 27, 165, 173, 183-4
  dosages 194
L. casei 29, 184
L. caucasicus (*L. kefir*) 29, 184
L. delbrueckii 29, 184
L. plantarum 29, 184
L. salivarius 29, 184
L. thermophilus 173
Lappe, Prof. Marc 18-19, 45, 66, 72, 154-5, 169-70, 209
laxatives, during fasts 113, 115

'leaky bowel' 156, 157, 160, 166, 187-8
Legionnaire's disease 50
Lewis, Dr. Doug 141
licorice 135-6, 163
lifestyle changes 102, 106-10
lincomycin 50, 73, 155
lincosamides 50, 73-5
linseed 115, 165
liver disease 83, 86, 168-9, 188
lunch, as part of immune-enhancement 125
lupus 187
lymph nodes 95
lymphocytes 94-6

McKenna, Dr. John 12
MacPherson, Dr. 156
macrolides 49-50, 75-7, 82
macrophages 94, 95, 96
magnesium 130-1
Malaleuca alternifolia 137
manganese 131
massage 109
mast cells 96
mastic gum 181
MDR-TB 39
ME *see* chronic fatigue syndrome
meditation 109
meningitis 30
menopausal problems 174-5, 188-9
menstrual problems 174-5
metronidazole 78-9
  side-effects 78-9, 84, 86
Micrococcus luteus 170

and TSS 160
S. epidermis 7, 31
S. haemolyticus 31
stealth bacteria 53
steroids 98
stimulant drugs 99
storage, of probiotics 192
Streptococcus faecalis 28-9, 184
S. faecium 28, 184
S. pneumoniae 32
S. thermophilus 28, 184
Streptomycaes griseus 46
streptomycin 46, 66, 68
stress 190
    and acne 172
    factors 107
    and immune function 99,
        108-9
Stretch, Eileen 160
sugar, in diet 97
sugar-loading test 158
sulfa antibacterial drugs *see*
    sulfonamides
Sulfacetamide 59
sulfanilamide 41
sulfapyridine 41
sulfonamides 34, 41, 59-61
    side-effects 59-61, 84
sulfur drugs 40-4, 56-7
superantigens:
    byproduct of superbugs 8
    and childhood eczema 7
superbugs:
    evolution 8
    in HAI 2
supplementation:

during antibiotic treatment 193,
    195-6, 203, 205-6
during fast 113
for babies 203-6
to enhance immune system
    126-33
symbiosis 24, 57
symptoms:
    of CFS 161, 167
    prior to CFS or FMS 162, 168
    of weakened immune system
        100-1
    of yeast overgrowth 157-8
synthetic antibacterial substances
    56-7
systemic action 56

T-lymphocytes (T-cells) 94-6
TB 38-9
tea tree oil 137
temafloxacin 84
terramycin 48
tetracycline 18, 34, 70, 169-70
tetracyclines 47-9, 70-3
    side-effects 48-9, 83, 85
Thermo Regulatory Hydrotherapy
    (TRH) 143-7
thrombophlebitis 84
thrush *see* Candida overgrowth
thymus gland 95, 99
Toxic Shock Syndrome (TSS) 30-1,
    160
toxicity:
    antibiotic 82-7
    environmental 98, 201-2
    selective 58

treatment, difficulties 52-4
tretinoin 170
trimethoprim 60
TSS *see* Toxic Shock Syndrome
tuberculosis 38-9

ulcers 180-1
upsets, to friendly bacteria 185-6
use, of antibiotics, criteria for 87-8,
  92, 196-7
Usnea barbata 137

vaccinations, and immune
  function 99
vaginal area, candidiasis 160
vancomycin 31, 32, 50
  side-effects 50, 85, 86
vegetable broth 115-16
vegetable juice 111, 116
viral infections:
  hyperthermic therapy 141
  inappropriate treatment 13, 87,
    210
visualization 102, 109

vitamin A 127
vitamin BU1u 132
vitamin BU2u 132
vitamin BU5u 133
vitamin BU6u 127, 133
vitamin BU12u 133
vitamin B complex 132-3
vitamin C 127, 128-9
vitamin E 127, 129

white blood cell, improving
  function 150
white blood cell count, probiotic
  supplementation for 194
wrong use 12-13, 87-8

yeast die-off 166
yeast overgrowth *see* Candida
  overgrowth
yeast-based foods 164, 166
yoghurt, live 122, 172-3

zinc 127, 130, 171